In ancient times, the Chinese developed the magnetic compass, which provided a new way for people to understand direction, and gunpowder, with which man could harness power. Today, it is time to present to the world the theory of Macro-Corelationism, which utilizes a Three Dimensional Four Inter-Channel model with which the flow of Qi in the body can be better understood. The use of Qi Gong to harness power, important both for health maintenance and healing, is also discussed here.

- An adaptation of acupuncture theory to conditions in the modern Western world.

- New interpretation of Yin/Yang theory and Five Element theory.

- It is not difficult to learn how to do diagnosis and prognosis of cancer and other diseases. Many cancers of the reproductive organs are not caused by the intake of environmental carcinogens or by genetic inheritance. Instead, they can be caused by lower back problems involving the spine, or by blockages of Qi energy through the 5th toe (Urinary Bladder Channel) or the 4th toe (Gall Bladder Channel connecting to the Liver Channel).

- Learn to build Qi energy.

- An assignment to scientists and doctors for the 21st century: Observe animals and survey your patients using the Three Dimensional Four Inter-Channel model in order to understand Qi energy and its relationship to disease.

- Western medicine, for all its advances in technology and microscopic analysis, has limitations which are inherent in specialization and laboratory testing. As we near the dawn of the new millennium, it is time to include Myung Kim's theory of Macro-Corelationism in our understanding of the workings of the human body.

ABOUT THE AUTHOR

Myung Chill Kim was born in Korea in 1942. He is the seventh child in a family of eleven brothers and sisters and has lived with Oriental martial arts and Oriental Medicine for his entire life. He is the 37th generation Doctor of Oriental Medicine.

He moved to the United States in 1970. His first book, "Acupuncture for Self Defense" was published in 1971. This book deals with acupuncture or pressure points to paralyze or heal an opponent.

He performed acupuncture anesthesia in June of 1973 at the Naval Hospital at Portsmouth, Virginia.

Myung Chill Kim graduated from New York City Technical College in 1981 with a degree in biology. He also graduated from the Emperor's College of Oriental Medicine in 1984 and received his degree of Doctor of Oriental Medicine in 1988 from Samra University of Oriental Medicine.

He discovered the main causative factor of cancer by applying his martial art and acupuncture channel theory developed through his clinical research of acupuncture and herbal medicine in the United States for the last 26 years.

Currently, Myung Chill Kim practices acupuncture and herbal medicine in Cambridge, Massachusetts. He is currently writing books on Qi Gong, Herbal Medicine and Martial Arts which will be published over the next few years.

ORIENTAL MEDICINE AND CANCER
(Macro -Corelationism)

By Myung Chill Kim

FIRST EDITION
SEVEN GALAXY PUBLICATION^{T.M.}

DEDICATION

This book is dedicated to the memory to Tae S. Kim, my father, and to my Taoist ancestors. Also, to my mother whose unique knowledge of Oriental Medicine and support made this book possible.

Copyright © 1996 by Myung Chill Kim

All rights reserved. No part of this book may be reproduced without the author's written permission.

Published by:
Seven Galaxy Publication ™, PO Box 330, Belmont, MA 02178

First Printing 1997 • Printed in the Korea

Library of Congress Cataloging in Publication Data.
Library of Congress Catalog Card Number 96-92634
Oriental Medicine and Cancer / by Myung Chill Kim
First Edition. Includes bibliographical references and index
ISBN 1-890016-00-4 $19.95

ACKNOWLEDGMENTS

I would like to express my appreciation to the following friends, Mark Mills and Michael Kopel, without whose rigorous writing and typing efforts this book would never have come to be. Also, my thanks to Chris Edwards, Francis Scholtz, and Bobie Flynn for their writing efforts and to Francis and Debby Lang for their research. My thanks also goes to Master Chen Yo Yu for his Chinese calligraphy. Most drawings were beautifully done by Elisa Bernstein and other drawings were done by Roger Levin. My thanks also goes to Sandra Rich for her computer graphic design, Kevin Dacey for the photography, to Pam Summa for her editing, to Lisa Allen for her drawing and beautiful glass acupuncture model, to Sue Macy for her proof-reading and Jeffrey Grossman for book design and cover design.

Finally, I would like to thank my wife Sung Chu, John, Stella and family members for their continued support.

WARNING - DISCLAIMER

This book is intended to provide information on general theory of Oriental Medicine and how to diagnose, prognose and treat cancer with Oriental Medicine.

The theories of Oriental Medicine discussed in this book were adopted to allow for the differences between the Western and Eastern lifestyles. It is intended for the use of laymen as well as acupuncturists and other medical practitioners. Western medical theory is not discussed here nor will you learn about acupuncture points and how to find them.

This book should only be used as a general guide and should not be considered the best source of information on cancer but as a new approach to cancer.

The author and Seven Galaxy Publication shall have neither liability nor responsibility to any person or organization with respect to any mental or physical damage caused directly or indirectly by the information in this book. For a full refund, you may return this book, with the original receipt, in good condition to the publisher within a week of purchase. The book must be properly packed as it was when you received it by mail.

Table of Contents

Introduction

"Gentlemen and Ladies"

"I have traveled around the eastern, western, southern, and northern parts of the United States."

In order to understand Oriental Medicine, Westerners must open their minds to the vast differences between Eastern and Western ways of thinking. There are profound differences in orientation, approaches to movement, ways in which language is used to refer to movement in nature, and the perception of how human beings are related to nature.

People in American, European, Arabic, and Indian cultures think about direction in the following sequence: North, South, East, and West. Western culture is characterized by movement and exploration. The herding of cattle through wild grasslands, the caravans crossing vast deserts in search of food and water, the sailing of ships in search of new lands and new opportunities for trade, and the voyages through space in pursuit of knowledge about the universe — these restless movements of the Western mind are perhaps guided by the use of the Northern star as a point of orientation. In Taoist terms, we would say that as a culture of movement, the West is Yang.

In Eastern culture, in contrast, Chinese and Korean people orient according to: East, West, South, and North. People have been tempered by thousands of years of agriculture. The orientation towards life and health is based on farming, literally cultivating "what is." Relative to the West we could be called a Yin culture. When Koreans sleep, they point their heads towards the East or South. As you will learn in this book, Qi Gong and other forms of meditation also recommend facing East and South. The rising of the sun and its heating of the earth influenced the livelihood of our ancestors so much that we still use it as a basis for orienting our lives.

The Chinese, Mongols, and Tibetans have basic directional orientations that they use in daily living. In China, the dead are displayed in their houses during mourning in coffins with their heads facing north or the deceased is buried facing north under ground; this tradition has been adapted by Koreans. Mongols, like Koreans, build their houses facing South to take advantage of the sun's light and heat since their weather can be extremely cold.

Another example illustrating the differences in orientation between the West and the East is the compass. The Chinese originally invented the magnetic compass, called the Chi Nan Jen - Chi meaning pointing; Nan meaning South and Jen meaning needle. Westerns assumed, when they recreated the compass for their use, that the magnetic direction was north. Once again, we see the clear cut difference in orientation.

We can also see differences in orientation between Asians and Westerners by looking at their vacation preferences. When Asian people vacation in Hawaii, they use Oahu Island, where Honolulu, Waikiki beach, and Pearl Harbor are located, as their base camp. They may visit the other four islands within one day, one island at a time, but they return to their base camp at Oahu each night. In contrast, European-Americans and other Caucasian-Americans usually stay on one island for a few days before moving onto the next island.

Asians and Caucasians also express their different orientations to life by the way they spend their money. When Asian-Americans become wealthy, they tend to buy large mansions and luxury cars. But wealthy, action-oriented Americans use their money to purchase horses, large yachts, and jet airplanes in addition to their houses and cars.

The Chinese refer to the lunar calendar as a Yin calendar and to the solar calendar as a Yang calendar. The Chinese primarily used the Yin calendar until the 19th century, when China and India were colonized by the Europeans. Since then, they have used both. Although China, along with Korea and other Asian countries, celebrates New Year's day according to both calendars, the Chinese and Koreans still favor the New Year's day on the Yin (lunar) calendar.

Differences in orientation between West and East are also reflected in their respective approaches to science and medicine. Western science developed through the use of lenses in microscopes and telescopes to observe the very small and the very distant. In contrast, Oriental science developed through close observation of what was directly experienced. Meditation and understanding of the flow of Qi energy in the body were the keys to this kind of knowledge.

Oriental science and philosophy looked at everything in context with everything else, instead of dividing, separating, and analyzing parts. During the Tang Dynasty in China (618 A.D. - 907 A.D.), a Taoist writer expressed this connectedness in a poem:

"Dear Creator, why did you create not only human beings but also mosquitoes, flies, spiders, and other insects that harm people?" Said the Creator: "You stupid human! This world is for everybody. It is not only for human beings!" In response, a Taoist stuck his hand through a hole in the mosquito net to share his blood with the insects.

The main functions of Oriental Medicine are to open Qi stagnations in the body and to revitalize body functions by understanding how body systems are interconnected. The doctor heals by restoring the body to its natural condition in its environment.

The Western medical tradition has made great contributions through its tradition of dissection, analysis, and the development of diagnostic tools to detect diseases. But the emphasis on tearing apart and destroying has its limits. We see this with the overuse of drugs to kill germs, kill pains and kill parasites. Similarly, the Western political policy of dividing and conquering in war has broken up Asian and Arabic nations and families. In Oriental tradition, the victors in warfare respected the integrity of conquered nations and their families.

The Western tradition of analysis and separation has led to specialization in its approach to medical care. Specialties such as surgery, internal medicine, ophthalmology, pediatrics, gynecology, and psychiatry focus on small parts of the human body with the attempt to kill the source of disorder in these parts. Oriental Medicine treats the entire condition of the body, not simply the disease, by combining all of the symptoms that appear in the patient to discern patterns of disorder and lack of harmony.

Where Western medicine tends to see disease or syndrome as having a single cause, Oriental medical theory looks at a wide variety of causes for a single health problem. Constipation is a good example of a very common condition with many different causes. At this point the terms and concepts which appear below may be unfamiliar to you, but they will become clearer as you read further along in the book.

CONSTIPATION

1) EXCESS TYPES

A. Heat in Yang Ming Channels (Stomach and Large Intestine)
Abdominal pain and/or distention
Tidal fever in morning
Profuse sweating, thirst, scanty urine
Mouth ulcers
Tongue — Red body with dry, thick yellow coat
Pulse — Slippery, full
Seen during fevers and other acute febrile diseases.

B. Liver/Spleen Qi Stagnation

Fullness in the chest
Breast distention
Easily angered
Nausea, vomiting
Headache
Tongue — Pink with a white or sticky white coat
Pulse — Wiry or wiry and deep
Triggered by emotional stress obstructing the smooth flow of Qi.

2) DEFICIENCY TYPES

A. Lung/Spleen Qi Deficiency
Constipation with soft stool
Difficulty in passing stool (Due to muscle weakness)
Shortness of breath
Fatigue, tiredness
Low voice

Organ prolapse
Pale face
Cold extremities
Tongue — Pale with a thin white coat or swollen with teeth marks
Pulse —- Soft and weak

B. Kidney/Spleen Yang Deficiency
Dark facial color
Cold extremities
Preference for warmth
Profuse urination
Nocturia
Tongue —- Pale with a white coat
Pulse —- Deep and small

C. Blood and Yin Deficiency
Much difficulty in eliminating stool
Dry mouth
Palpitations
Pale lips and nails
Tongue —- Pale or red with no coating
Pulse —- Thready and rapid or forceless

When treating constipation with acupuncture, some points will be the same to move the stagnation in the intestines and some will be different to address different underlying causes. However, when treating constipation with herbal medicine, the formulas will be very different, unless the patient is being given laxatives. For instance, excess type constipation is treated with purgative herbs and deficiency type with moistening herbs.

TRADITIONAL CHINESE MEDICINE AND CONTEMPORARY AMERICAN SOCIETY

The life style of a Chinese farmer has not changed dramatically over the past thousand years. There have been some technological advances and certainly there is better access to health care, but the basic conditions of life and work are similar. Thus the health problems described in the medical classics closely resemble those faced by a contemporary doctor of Traditional Chinese Medicine. However, if this doctor were to come to the United States to speak, the doctor might find that the lecture did not fit as well with the contemporary American situation.

TODAY IN THE UNITED STATES WE SEE:

- More mental stress
- Labor involving machinery
- Auto accident-related injuries
- Gunshot wounds
- Sports addiction (Over-exercise)
- Emotional trauma resulting from broken family life, abuse, etc.
- Damage to the ear, including partial loss of hearing, due to vibra tions from loud music
- Surgical scarring
- Cancer
- Drug problems
- Heavy emphasis on competition on the job, in sports, etc.
- Dietary problems like anorexia, bulimia, and resulting malnutrition
- Bodily harm from popular, dangerous sports such as sky diving, rock climbing, parachuting, bungee jumping, white water rafting, race car driving, boxing and football.

These modern American health problems are not directly discussed in the Chinese medical classics and require modern approaches. Since the United States is a nation with life styles, cultures, and dietary habits radically different from those of China, the practice of Oriental Medicine in the United States must necessarily diverge somewhat from that practiced in China today.

But Oriental Medicine can be adapted for people who live in modern industrialized countries. This book has been written to show how different Oriental medical theories can fit the health problems that plague Americans at the end of the Twentieth Century and into the Twenty First Century.

Chapter 1

A Taoist Monk

Shortly before dawn on a late autumn morning, a middle-aged man came walking along a narrow country road towards a small village. The dried grass in the fields and the harvested rice paddies at the side of the road were covered with white frost that gleamed in the light from the moon which was setting over the western mountains. As the man approached to within a mile of the village, he heard the cawing of a crow and the barking of a fox and paused. He looked ahead towards the entrance to the village and breathed deeply, smelling the air. Then he said to himself, "There is an old lady in this village who is dying from kidney disease. And somewhere else close by an old dog is dying."

The man then walked the last mile to the edge of the village, where he paused once more to look around and smell the air. Afterwards he approached a small hut where white smoke curled up out of a thin chimney.

"Is anybody home?" he called out.

A young woman emerged from the kitchen door rubbing her eyes sleepily. She looked at the man standing in the cold and replied "Who are you and what can I do for you?"

"I have just come down from the mountains. I believe that there is an old woman here who is very sick and I would like to help her."

The young woman invited him inside, where indeed there was an old woman. She was huddled on the floor of the small hut and breathing very shallowly. She seemed to be nearing death.

The Taoist[1] monk, for that is who he was, removed one silver acupuncture needle from the upper pocket of his jacket. He thrust the needle towards her hands, feet and chest without actually piercing her skin. He then set his silver needle down on the floor and shook his hands over her body, again without touching her, in order to put Qi[2] energy into her body. After this he rolled the woman on to her side and again took up his silver needle, thrusting it towards her waist and scapular areas, after which he again moved his hands over her as he had done before.

The old woman began to feel stronger. She opened her eyes and raised herself up to look at the man standing beside her. "You must be a Taoist master," she said. "I appreciate what you have done for me by saving me from death. I now have one more request for you. I need to live at least fifteen more days. My son is traveling to a country market and it will take him that long to return. And I hope to see him again before I die."

The Taoist told her daughter-in-law, for that is who the younger woman was, that she should wash the older woman's hands and feet with warm water three times a day. This would ensure that she would survive until her son's return.

He then walked out of the house and passed through the village as the sky began to grow light just before sunrise. He sniffed the air once more and then walked to another house where he found a dog lying outside, unable to even raise its head at his approach. He waved his palms over the dog to give it Qi energy. The dog then slowly rose and shook itself, cocked its head, looked at the Taoist monk and began to wag its tail. It then barked in a very low voice.

The Taoist smiled and replied, "It was nothing. Don't mention it." He bent down and stroked the dog's head and then straightened and walked on again.

As he neared the far end of the village, he noticed a tall tree growing next to a large rock. On one of the branches of the tree the needles were turning brown and beginning to drop off, so he stood before it and put Qi into the tree branch. He then studied the rock and thought to himself, "This rock's color is not very good," and for good measure gave Qi to the rock. And then he left the village and continued on his way to his unknown destination.

How had the Taoist realized that the old woman and the dog were dying before he even entered their village? When the fox barked and the crow cawed, traditional Korean villagers saw it as an omen that someone was about to die. But what is the real reason for these beliefs? It is not that these animals have psychic powers but that they possess highly evolved physical abilities. Both of these animals are scavengers with highly developed olfactory senses that allow them to detect the smell of decay in dying creatures.

The Taoist, having spent much time in the wilds observing nature, could listen to the communications of animals and know whether they were calling to their mate or protecting their territory, whether they were in danger or had found food. Even you, the reader, can probably listen to dogs barking in the distance and tell whether they are playing, fighting or barking at strangers. The Taoists, with their heightened perceptions, can hear much more than an average human and are even able to understand the meanings of many different animal calls. Like many animals, they are also able to detect scents at great distances.

The Taoist monk was in a state of heightened sensory awareness. He had been fasting, meditating and practicing Qi Gong in a cave in the mountains for the previous 100 days. (Although rare today, this kind of Taoist practice was more common in Korea about 100 years ago.) When he had finished his 100 days of solitude he emerged from the cave and made his way down from the mountains where he passed through this village.

The world's greatest spiritual leaders, men like Buddha, Moses, Jesus Christ, Mohammed, and the ancient Taoist monks, all practiced similar forms of fasting meditation during their lives for 30, 40 or even 100 days at a time. Even today on the outskirts of Beijing, China, there are military special forces training schools where trainees fast in caves for twenty-one days, learning Qi Gong meditation and sharpening their perceptual skills.

North Korean spies are also trained in this way, which enables them to feel the presence of humans or even small animals like rabbits in the darkness at a distance of 100 meters. Using only this special technique developed through meditation, their senses are so acute that they can detect buried land mines. With these skills they can infiltrate the heavily guarded border between North and South Korea.

But within two years after coming to the South, these spies can lose the ability to use their special training and they may even find that their normal sensory functions like hearing, sight, and smell have become impaired. This is due to the fact that they can no longer continue the Taoist Qi Gong meditation that they had practiced in the mountains of North Korea.

During the war in Viet Nam, it was very difficult to capture Viet Cong officers. Many had been trained at the military special forces training school near Beijing where they learned martial arts and Ninja [3] skills. When pursued they knew how to hide under water and breathe through reeds. They could also plaster themselves with mud and leaves and lie motionless to camouflage themselves when they were in danger of detection.

Yet they sometimes met their match in the South Korean Tiger troops. The South Koreans were forbidden to use any substances containing scents, from coffee and cigarettes to deodorant and toothpaste, which might give a clue to their presence. When they hid in ambush they not only caught Viet Cong soldiers but were actually able to hunt and kill approaching tigers. What sort of training must these Tiger troops have had to be able to successfully apprehend the Viet Cong?

Martial arts movies have become very popular over the years and by now probably everyone is familiar with Ninjas from Japanese samurai movies or their equivalents in Chinese and Korean films. They camouflage their faces with black cloth and cover their bodies with black suits. Then they infiltrate their enemies' strongholds on espionage or assassination missions. Sometimes they are shown communicating to each other while they are in hiding without being heard by the other people in the room. This is not simply a cinematic device. Someone who has received true Ninja training has developed auditory skills much sharper than those of ordinary humans. Like many animals they are able to hear sounds of much lower frequencies than the average person.

Using their heightened senses they are also able to detect from a distance how many of their enemies are in hiding, whether outdoors in a forest or on the other side of a thick wall. They are even able to see the spirits of dead people and ghosts. Training to develop such extraordinary skills originated in India, Tibet, and China long ago, and was exported to Japan via Korea.

In 1948, when I was six years-old, my family escaped from North Korea. All together we were ten brothers and sisters as well as my parents. Life in the North had become impossible for us since the

Communists had come to power. My oldest sister was the first to attempt to escape. But the Communists sank the boat in which she was sailing to the South and she was drowned. Her body washed ashore in what was then a part of South Korea and my father later visited the area and found the grave. It now lies on the North Korean side of the border and no one from my family has visited it for many years.

The next group to leave consisted of two older brothers, a friend and an uncle. My parents, an older brother and sister, a younger brother, and I made up the third group. We hid in houses during the day and walked all night. We were led by guides, each of whom had his own section of the mountains with which he was familiar. These guides were paid well for their dangerous job.

We were traveling during the full moon, so that we could have been seen even in the middle of the night. At one point on the trip, our guide slowed his steps and looked into the distance. He then told us "Someone is fishing in the lake up ahead. It must be a Communist guard." None of us were able to see into the distance like the guide, so we could see nothing but the forest and shadows, but we froze in our tracks at his words.

Because of this danger we had to remain where we were until the guard had tired of fishing and left the lake shore. We hid for more than two hours. I remember that my baby brother cried and my father coughed even though they tried as hard as they could to muffle the sounds. We knew that the guides had extraordinarily acute senses and they sometimes took off their rice straw sandals and walked barefoot so that they made even less sound as they walked. Their feet were as hard as an animal's.

The Viet Cong against whom I fought in the jungles of Viet Nam also had very sharp senses and reactions as quick as the other creatures of the forest. If I could take some of these Viet Cong soldiers and the Korean mountain people who served as guides and go off to a cave and practice fasting Qi Gong meditation for 21 days, I am sure that they would develop abilities like those of the Taoist at the beginning of this chapter.

Oriental Medicine is much different than Western medicine and very different diagnostic methods and abilities are employed when examining patients. Even within Oriental Medicine the techniques used to detect disease vary widely. One practitioner can diagnose a patient perfectly just by looking at the patient and smelling the odor emanating from the body. Another might base the diagnosis solely on information gained by abdominal palpation. Some Taoists are able to see inside the human body with their extraordinary visual power obtained through fasting Qi Gong meditation. But most doctors of Oriental Medicine check the pulse and look at the tongue of the patient and complete their diagnosis by asking questions about the patient's condition.

Some practitioners of Oriental Medicine are able to put Qi into a patient through an acupuncture needle which does not touch the patient's skin, like the Taoist mentioned earlier. Others simply touch the patient with the needle but do not penetrate the skin and are able in this way to transmit Qi.

Most acupuncturists, however, do insert the needle into the patient's body. Some are able to put Qi into a patient in this manner, but most ordinary practitioners can only open channels where Qi has stagnated.

When the Taoist healer visited the village where the old woman was ill, he was able to deduce a few things about her prognosis. He knew that she was in a serious state which was worsening due to the change of season. This was especially true because she was suffering from a Kidney problem and such conditions will become more severe with the onset of winter and cold weather.

He advised the old woman's daughter-in-law to wash her hands and feet with warm water, which is a basic Taoist treatment method. This helps Qi to circulate evenly throughout the body. Taoists always rub their hands and feet vigorously before and after meditation or Qi Gong practice to ensure smooth circulation of Qi.

Some of my patients have taken my advice and put their hands and feet in warm water for five to ten minutes every day and they have been very happy with the results. I would suggest that my readers apply this warm water treatment themselves and see whether they observe any changes in their own condition.

I understand that many acupuncturists insert needles into a point on the sole of the foot (Kidney 1/Yongquan)[4] or on the palm of the hand (Pericardium 8/Laogong)[5] when the patient feels dizzy or faints during an acupuncture or moxa[6] treatment. I believe that this can actually make the condition worse by shocking the patient with pain, as the palms and soles are the parts of the body most sensitive to pain.

There is another important reason to avoid needling a patient's palms and soles. This is the potential risk of infection. The palm probably comes into contact with more germs than any other part of the body during the day, and even at night we can scratch other parts of ourselves in our sleep. Infections, should they arise, are much slower to heal on the palms and soles compared to the dorsum of the foot or back side of the hand. So instead of needling the sole or the palm I would advise using the warm water treatment.

The soles of the feet are also very susceptible to Qi and Blood stagnation because of the gravitational force of the Earth. They also tend to perspire easily due to poorly ventilated shoes. Even when young and healthy people get an infection on the soles of their feet they sometimes do not heal properly. Occasionally they never heal and surgery to remove the infected area is the result. When antibiotics fail to control the infection, it can recur again and again.

I have seen many young and healthy people who have lost a foot or been amputated further up the leg at the ankle, the knee or even higher. These amputations have been the result of motorcycle accidents, injuries incurred during the War in Viet Nam, or, tragically, because of infections that did not heal properly.

Some diabetics, once they develop a foot infection, have to suffer progressive amputations all the way up to the groin area. I believe that if diabetics practice Qi Gong and/or receive appropriate acupuncture treatment that this can be prevented. At the very least, they should be sure to put their hands and feet in warm to hot water many times per day to stimulate Qi and Blood circulation in their bodies.

Children sometimes develop hiccups when they come into contact with cold air after they have eaten or when they drink cold liquids immediately after heavy physical exertion, especially when they are wet from sweating. In America, parents want to give their children water to drink to stop their hiccups. But this is actually another situation where the warm water treatment would be more helpful.

If someone has indigestion, do not try to warm the stomach area with a hot pad or a hot towel. This will only make the condition worse. Instead immerse the hands and feet in warm to hot water. Then massage the lumbar area of the lower back, just an inch or so above the waist. You will find a tender spot there, which is Urinary Bladder 21/Weishu[7], the Back Shu[8] Point of the Stomach. When this point is massaged, the patient's pale face and bluish lips will both turn red.

In the 1960s Korean scientists performed experiments in which they immersed animals' four feet in hot water. When the blood flow in the stomach area was measured a few minutes later it was found to have increased. Later blood flow through their entire bodies increased.

But when you use the warm water treatment be sure to only immerse your hands and feet in the water. If you soak your whole body in the bathtub you will feel better but your indigestion or other Qi stagnation conditions will not improve. Soaking only the hands and feet can even help in an emergency situation. In my experience this has worked for fainting, heat stroke, heart attack, epidemic fever and even when a patient is near death. A few months ago, a nurse who was one of my Qi Gong students helped a kidney dialysis patient who fainted while she was on duty by immersing his hands and feet in warm water. The patient soon revived. Two years ago a 16 year-old boy visited my clinic with diarrhea and a mysterious fever. His body temperature ranged between 102° and 104° and his head felt quite hot. His mother told me that he suffered this condition many times a year but that no doctor of western medicine had been able to help him. They probably applied an ice pack directly to his head to try to cool him down.

Even though he had a fever I gave him a warm water treatment. Three minutes after immersing his hands and feet his fever began to go down and five minutes after I had inserted acupuncture needles he began to feel better. He was fully recovered after receiving three treatments in a week. The following year he returned with the same problem. This time I treated him twice and he recovered. Since then

I have not heard from him.

Three years ago, a woman brought her 60 year-old mother into my clinic for acupuncture treatment. She was suffering from severe emotional distress, depression, nervousness, and sensitivity to pain. Even before I inserted any needles in her she was almost in a panic state, breathing shallowly and rapidly. So I gave her a warm water treatment and afterwards gave her acupuncture. After the needles were withdrawn I again had her wash her hands with warm water. She felt very relaxed and has continued to give herself warm water treatments every day.

If you are faced with a stressful situation, like a court battle, licensing exam, a tennis or boxing match, or even if you have only eaten a light dinner and are experiencing some form of indigestion or nervous stomach, try giving yourself a warm water treatment and do some breathing exercises. I think you will be pleased with the results. If people in this world applied warm water treatments, they could probably save at least one quarter of their present medical expenses.

Where warm water is not available, say in an emergency situation, you should rub the patients hands and feet with your hands to warm them. Another waterless method is to apply moxa to Large Intestine 4/Hegu[9] (between the thumb and forefinger) and Liver 3/Taichong[10] (between the big and second toes).

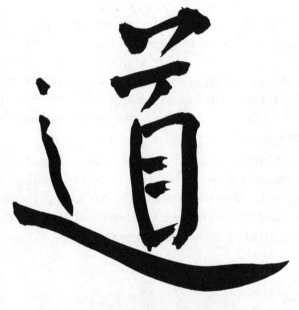

TAO (DAO)

Chapter 2

How To Develop Qi
(Internal Energy)

I have been teaching in the United States since my arrival in 1970. To learn meditation, Qi Gong[11,] Tai Chi[12], martial arts or Oriental Medicine, students must be willing to devote the time and effort necessary to learn these arts. But the following three methods of breathing have been developed for easy learning so that people can gain some benefit and get a taste of Qi for themselves. Before practicing any of these exercises, rub your hands and feet for a few moments until they feel warm. Also keep in mind these guidelines.

General Guidelines for Qi Gong Practice:

- Face either east or south.
- Practice at least one hour before or after eating.
- Do not practice if you are overly tired, hungry, sick, or emotionally upset.
- Qi Gong practice should leave one feeling calm and centered. Consult a Qi Gong master if you feel excessively joyful or sad after practicing.
- Ideally, practice twice a day at sunrise and noon.
- Do not practice at night before you go to sleep. It is best to have at least four hours between Qi Gong practice and going to bed.
- Practice in a quiet, clean place and wear loose fitting clothes.
- Breathe in and out through your nose deeply and slowly. Imagine your breath to be a fine continuous silken thread. Or breathe like a newborn baby taking a nap. Beginning students should do a short breathing cycle, inhaling for a count of five and exhaling for a count of ten. More advanced students will naturally do a longer cycle, perhaps inhaling for a count of ten and exhaling for a count of twenty, or even longer.

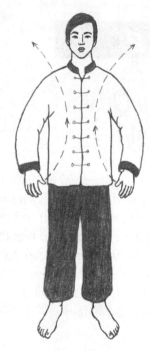

Figure 2A-1

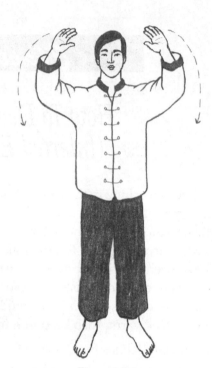

Figure 2A-2

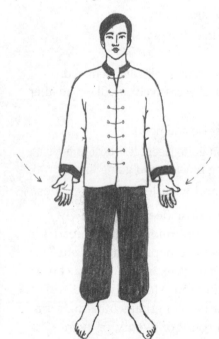

Figure 2A-3

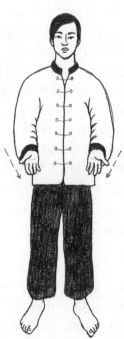

Figure 2A-4

- Never combine Qi Gong with weight lifting exercises or practice when you are intoxicated.

- Pregnant women should avoid these exercises.

- If you develop nausea, vomiting, a headache, or insomnia from Qi Gong practice, do the tension relief breathing exercises described below. Then immerse your hands and feet in warm water for ten minutes.

QI GONG BREATHING

1. Touch the tip of the tongue to the roof of the mouth.

2. Inhale through the nose, drawing your breath down into your lower abdomen. Hold your breath for a few seconds and then exhale very slowly through the nose.   Exhalation should always be longer than inhalation.

A. TENSION RELIEF BREATHING EXERCISE

1. Look straight ahead and focus your attention on a spot on the wall slightly below eye level.

2. Turn your hands so that the backs are facing forwards as shown in Figure 2A-1.

3. Inhale deeply through your nose and draw your hands and forearms upward from your lower abdomen. Then rotate them outwards in a large circle. See Figures 2A-1, 2A-2, 2A-3.

4. Push your palms forward with fingertips pointing towards the earth and exhale through your mouth, making the sound "Ssshhh." Imagine that you are pushing out all your bad feelings, thoughts, and emotions along with your breath. See Figure 2A-4.

If you feel angry, depressed, sad, or otherwise emotionally troubled, do this breathing exercise rapidly at first and then gradually slow down your rate of breathing. Repeat 10 to 20 times until you feel calmer.

B. QI GONG BREATHING

You will want to use lower abdominal breathing, so focus your attention on a point one inch below the navel. This area is known as the Lower Dan Tien (Red Planting Field). It is the source of internal power. Touch the tip of your tongue to the roof of your mouth. Inhale and exhale slowly through your nose. One breathing cycle should consist of a 3-5 second inhalation with the lower abdomen rising, holding the breath for 2-4 seconds, and then a 4-6 second exhalation as the lower abdomen sinks. With practice, the breathing cycles can grow longer, with the same ratio between inhaling, holding, and exhaling. Beginners should practice this breathing for 5 minutes, and can gradually increase to 30 minutes or an hour.

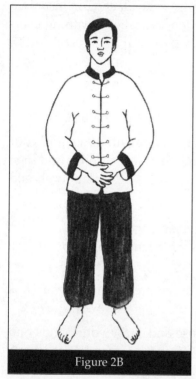
Figure 2B

The proper stance for this exercise should be natural and relaxed, with the feet as wide apart as the shoulders. Place the right hand over the Lower Dan Tien and cover the right hand with the left. A weak or disabled person can practice while seated on a chair or bed. (See Figure 2B for an illustration of the stance.)

As you practice, you may feel warmth on the stomach and saliva may collect in your mouth. These are good indications that Qi energy is building up. Swallow the accumulated saliva slowly, about one third of the volume with each swallow.

C. TAOIST CLOUD PUSHING BREATHING

1. In this exercise, the wrists should remain loose and the mind focused on the Lower Dan Tien. A relaxed, slow, floating feeling should be sought after.

2. Inhale and exhale through the nose.

3. Stand with your feet shoulder width apart. Hold your hands in front of your thighs with palms facing back. Inhale slowly. See Figure 2C-1.

4. As you inhale, slowly raise your hands with palms down, fin-

gers curved downward and elbows bent. See Figure 2C-2.

5. When your hands have reached shoulder height, exhale while extending your arms out to the side and turning your palms so that they are facing to the sides. Imagine that you are pressing white clouds in a blue sky. See Figure 2C-3.

6. Then hold your breath as you drop your arms slowly to the beginning position. Rest focused on the Lower Dan Tien for a moment before repeating. See Figure 2C-4.

7. Repeat at least 15 times. Then repeat while imagining the stored Qi energy in your Lower Dan Tien area rising up to your chest as you raise your arms. Then imagine the Qi energy radiating out through your palms as they are extended outward. After a few movements, you may begin to feel tingling and a warm sensation on your palms and fingertips. This is the sensation of Qi flow.

8. Close your eyes. Turn your hands so that the palms face each other as though you are holding a ball, keeping your elbows by your side. Move your hands slowly apart and together but do not touch them. You may feel that you are holding a "Qi Ball." Some people can even feel the pushing and pulling sensations of the electromagnetic wave force of Qi energy. If these three breathing exercises are practiced every day, you will sooner or later feel Qi energy yourself. See Figure 2C-5.

9. Straddle a chair with your legs apart and your stomach and chest facing the chair back. First, hold your hands above the chair back with the palms facing each other and move them closer and further apart, as shown in Figure 2C-6. Then rest the pinkie finger side of your wrists on the chair back as shown in Figure 2C-7. Try to feel the Qi sensation in both cases. As you compare the sensations you feel with these two movements, you can see how Qi flow can be easily blocked even by the slight interference of resting your wrists on the chair back.

10. Sit on a chair facing a partner. Both of you should extend your hands with the left palm facing up and the right palm facing down. Place your right palm above your partner's left and your left palm below your partner's right palm. Close your

eyes, touch the tip of your tongue to the roof of your mouth and breath slowly through your nose about 100 times. Both of you will feel warmth and Qi movement. See figure 2C-8.

Generally, children, younger people, women and people who are sensitive will feel Qi more quickly than those who are weak, or big and muscular, or have surgery scars or have had a spinal injury. But those who have difficulty feeling Qi can feel it after a few acupuncture treatments.

The best time to practice any Qi Gong is after meditation and after having immersed your hands and feet in warm water for five minutes.

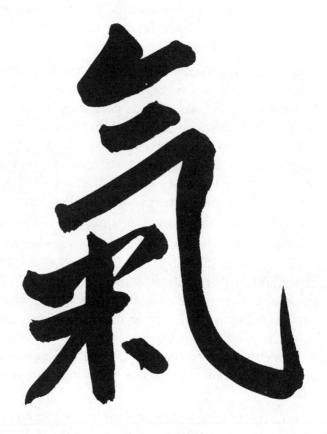

QI (CHI)

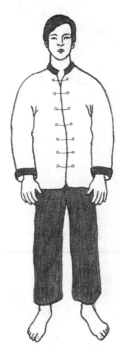

Figure 2C-1

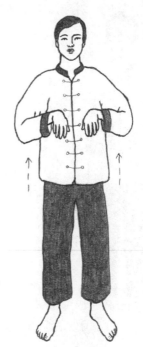

Figure 2C-2

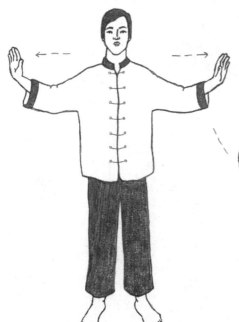

Figure 2C-3

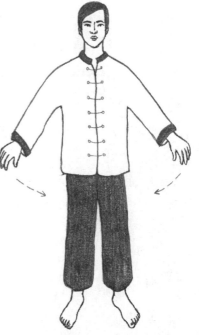

Figure 2C-4

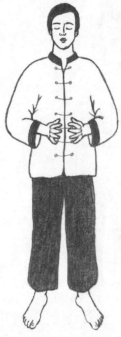

Figure 2C-5

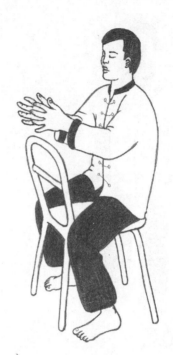

Figure 2C-6

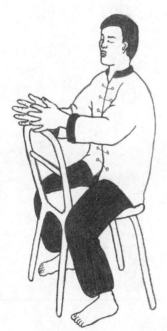

Figure 2C-7

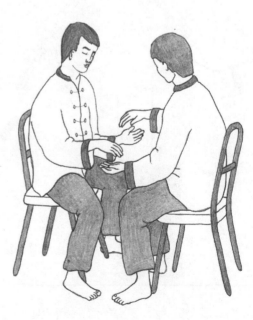

Figure 2C-8

Chapter 3
Qi, Jing, Xue, Shen, Hun, Po, Ling, & Body fluids

QI

To begin to feel Qi sensations in one's own body is one of the great steps towards self-realization.

The ancient Chinese believed that Qi was the fundamental basis of all matter and energy in the universe. Around the same time, the Hindus used the word "Prana" for a similar concept, the life force. The 2,000 year-old Chinese medical book *Nei Jing* (Internal Medicine) describes many different types of Qi which exist in the human body.

YUAN QI (SOURCE QI)

Inherited from parents and stored in the Kidneys. Its main function is reproduction. It is gradually depleted after age 40. The regular Japanese greeting "O Genki diska?" which means "How are you?" literally means "How is your Source Qi?"

YING QI (NUTRITIVE QI)

Comes from food and circulates through the vessels, supplying Qi to the internal organs. This is the Qi that is activated when an acupuncture needle is inserted.

WEI QI (DEFENSIVE QI)

Circulates over the surface of the body, protecting it from an external invasion of disease. It warms and nourishes the muscles and skin as it passes through them and also controls the opening and closing of the pores, regulating perspiration.

ZONG QI (ESSENTIAL QI)

Nourishes the Heart and Lungs which perform respiration.

QING QI (CLEAN QI)

Along with the supply of Source Qi available at birth, the body forms Clean Qi from the air and food it takes in.

Hopefully, many of the readers felt the Qi energy, the electromagnetic wave force in the human body, after practicing the exercises described in Chapter 2. From the moment that you first feel the flow of Qi in your body, you will begin to become more aware of your health and life style, your inner self and your relations with your surroundings and with the universe.

Many Asian people have believed that women should not conceive children on days when there are heavy rains, wind, and especially thunderstorms. It is thought that this could cause malformation of the fetus due to irregular Qi flow. Further, an expectant mother should not discuss, listen to, or even look at bad things.

JING

Jing, which is often translated as Essence, is divided into prenatal and postnatal aspects. Prenatal Jing is formed at conception from energies of one's parents, and could be considered to correspond to modern Western medical concepts like DNA[13], reproductive hormones and semen. Prenatal Jing determines a person's basic constitution. Postnatal Jing is formed after birth by Qi, which transforms food in the Stomach and Spleen.[14] Postnatal Jing is stored in the Kidneys.

Changes in the Jing over the course of life govern the development and changes of the body. The *Nei Jing* outlines the stages of physical development in a series of seven-year cycles for women and eight-year cycles for men.

Numerical cycles are considered significant in many Asian cultures. Both Koreans and Chinese celebrate the 100th day after a baby is born and the first birthday. In Japan the 210th day after a baby's birth is observed if the baby appears strong and healthy. Historically there were much higher rates of infant mortality in Asian countries, but these have been dramatically reduced by the introduction of Western immunization. Today the 100 and 210 day celebrations continue as traditions but the reason for celebrating these days has been lost.

After a child is born in Korea, it is customary to hang a straw rope in the door frame of the house. If the baby is a girl, charcoal is hung from the rope and if a boy, dried red peppers are used. The rope is left hanging for 21 days, allowing the mother to rest quietly and preventing germs from being carried into the house by non-family members.

BLOOD

Blood is formed from Kidney Jing and food. Blood helps in the production of Qi and the Qi moves the Blood. This may sound like a contradiction to the Western understanding that Blood is moved through the circulatory system by the pumping action of the heart. But Blood in Oriental Medicine is not exactly the same as the red fluid in the blood vessels. It is energetic as well as material in nature. You can observe after practicing Qi Gong movements that the palms of your hands have turned a mottled pink or even a red color due to the movement of Blood by your Qi.

This of course raises another question. If Qi moves Blood, what moves Qi? Qi does move of its own accord, but it can also be moved by your own will power. Much of Qi Gong practice involves the control and movement of Qi. Take for example, how the simple movement in which the arms are raised in a broad inward circular motion and the palms then press down moves Qi downwards (illustrated in Figures 3-1 to 3-4). Close your eyes and try doing this after the Qi Gong exercises described in Chapter 2. You may feel a tingling sensation in the soles of your feet when you do this, perhaps not the first time you try but certainly with enough practice. If you have a problem with one foot, you will feel it only in the other foot.

SHEN

Shen[15] is often translated as "spirit" in English. In East Asian countries, however, it is often translated as "God." Shen is stored in the Heart, and when the Heart Qi and Blood become deficient a person's thinking processes can be disturbed. Then such problems as poor memory, dull thinking and insomnia can result. Emotional problems such as depression and mental restlessness may also be seen in some cases. Conversely, emotional problems may themselves lead to deficiencies of Heart Qi and Blood with manifestations like palpitations and a weak or irregular pulse.

HUN, PO, LING

The Chinese Taoist philosopher Chuang Tzu (365-290 B.C.E.) said

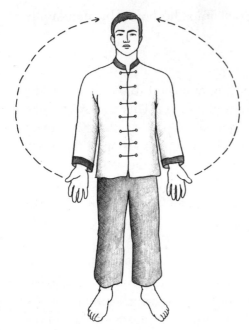

Figure 3-1

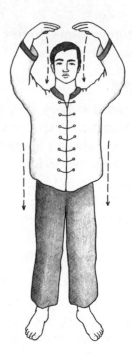

Figure 3-2

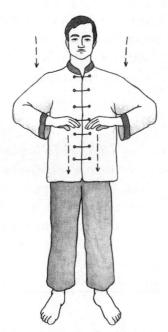

Figure 3-3

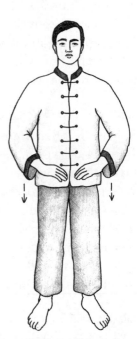

Figure 3-4

that death means that Qi has left the human body. Death can also be described as the permanent separation of Hun and Po from the body. Hun[16] is the Yang aspect of Qi which floats up to heaven when a person dies. It is rooted in the Liver and is associated with vitality and courage.

Po[17] is the Yin aspect of Qi. It is more physical than Hun and returns to the earth with the body after death. It is housed in the Lungs and is associated with the senses and the Essence as discussed earlier.

Ling[18] is what the Shen (Spirit) becomes after death.

BODY FLUIDS

The Chinese believed that the Small Intestine divided the body fluids into clear and turbid types. The clear fluids warm and nourish muscles and moisten the skin. The turbid fluids lubricate the joints and moisten the brain, spinal column and bone marrow. They also combine with the Nutritive Qi to form the Blood.

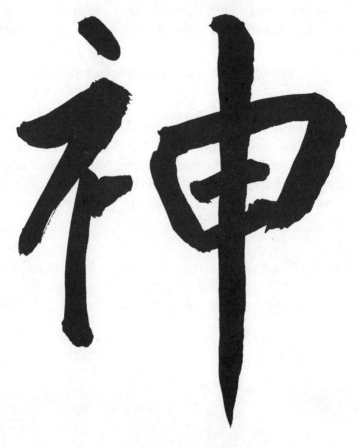

SHEN (SPIRIT)

Chapter 4

Causes of Disease

What causes disease? Another way to ask this question, I believe, is "What causes Qi stasis (stagnation)?"

Disease can be caused by many factors acting either separately or in conjunction with each other. These include the six exogenous factors, seven emotions, diet and nutrition, physical activity, scars and trauma, improper medical treatment, improper Qi Gong practice, astronomical influences, technological influences, infection, spirit possession, genetics, and stress.

SIX EXOGENOUS FACTORS

People who live in the temperate zones of this planet are more affected by seasonal changes than are people who live in either the tropics or the Arctic. I will explain this in more detail in Chapter Seven, Five Element Theory, where the relationships between seasons, the weather, climatic regions, and man's internal organs and emotions are discussed.

At the end of the Twentieth Century, we have more opportunities to travel longer distances than humans have ever had before.

In military life, younger soldiers suffer less when they are relocated from one region or country to another than the older soldiers do. The younger soldiers are able to adapt more quickly.

In the Winter of 1966, I returned home to Korea after having served in the Vietnam War. I practiced Cha Ryuk[19] (Korean hard style Qi Gong) and used herbal medicines to try to offset the stresses of moving from the tropics to a much more temperate climate. As a result, I did not experience any physical problems associated with regional change. I did, however, suffer from some mental instabilities. I was easily excitable and tense, which I attribute to the stress of living in a war zone and the difficulties of readjusting to a peacetime world.

I saw many of my comrades suffering from Cold even in the summer and from recurrences of the malaria that they had become infected with in Vietnam. I advised them to try acupuncture and herbal medicine instead of the modern cold pills that were popularly used to relieve the symptoms.

The six exogenous factors that can cause disease are Wind, Cold, Summer Heat, Dampness, Dryness, and Heat.

WIND

Wind usually attacks the upper part of the body, invading through the nose and mouth or passing through the neck area. It can accompany other factors such as Cold, Heat, and Damp. In these cases, Wind helps these factors to invade the body and to spread quickly. The Chinese names of acupuncture points like UB 10[20] (Wind Lake), which is located in the back of the neck below the occipital bone and lateral to the trapezius muscles, and UB 11[21] (Wind Gate), located about half an inch lateral to the first thoracic vertebra, reflect their usage in treating Wind-related problems.

Many office workers sit near the air conditioner, exposed to a cold wind all day long. This constant exposure makes them more susceptible to colds and flu, chronic muscle spasms, and headaches.

Pain which moves around (like common neuralgia) is called Wind Pain. This is differentiated from pain that remains fixed in one area, which is caused by Blood Stagnation.

In Chinese medicine there is another condition associated with Wind: paralysis.

COLD

When someone is exposed to cold temperatures for long periods of time they will lose both their body warmth and their Yang Qi. A Yang Deficiency Syndrome will be the result. (See Chapter 8 for a discussion of Yang Deficiency.)

Cold causes the arteries to constrict in order to conserve heat in the body. This causes disturbances in Qi flow.

SUMMER HEAT

Summer Heat occurs only as a result of exposure to extreme heat. It can injure Yin and deplete the Body Fluids. The most common manifestations of Summer Heat are fever and heavy sweating.

DAMPNESS

People who live in a damp environment due to the climate, work in damp surroundings, or even if they inhabit a basement apartment may find themselves feeling sluggish or heavy. Getting caught in the rain and having wet hair or clothes for too long, or eating or drinking too many cold liquids or food too rapidly, can create Cold Damp conditions, characterized by a heavy head, indigestion, nausea, and vomiting. A long-time vegetarian diet which emphasizes cold salads and fruit rather than balance can be another cause. It is easy to become a vegetarian if you live somewhere like India with a year-round hot climate. But people living in temperate zones with cold seasons, and even more so people living closer to the Poles, can easily become Yang Deficient and invaded by Cold-Damp.

Sometimes a person with low blood pressure will experience symptoms similar to those of Dampness: a feeling of heaviness, lethargy, indigestion or slow digestion, nausea and vomiting.

DRYNESS

During the autumn, dry air causes dry skin and dry lungs. This can lead to a dry cough and allergies and other lung problems. In the winter, home heating systems often produce extremely dry interior air.

One Arctic survival technique is to be sure to drink enough water to prevent dehydration. With insufficient fluid intake, the skin on the elbows and knees begins to dry and itch. When this occurs, it is recommended that people do not shower or bathe more than once or twice a week to prevent additional dehydration.

HEAT

Heat is different from Summer Heat. It can occur in any season. Sometimes there are warm spells in the winter, which are followed by outbreaks of influenza and other epidemic diseases. Heat can also be an occupational hazard. People who work near heat sources like ovens or blast furnaces will feel worse heat during the summer and much drier during the autumn. These sensations can be precursors to disease.

SEVEN EMOTIONS

The seven emotions are joy, anger, worry, over-thinking, sadness, fear and fright. We all feel these emotions constantly to one degree or another. Five Element Theory, which will be discussed in Chapter 7, holds that each emotion affects a different internal organ of the body. But all emotions also eventually affect the Heart, because the Heart is the house of the Shen or Spirit.

DIET AND NUTRITION

The Stomach receives food and the Spleen transforms it into Qi and Blood, so these two organs are the most affected by diet. Malnutrition weakens the Spleen and causes Qi and Blood to be Deficient. In the West, over-eating is a greater problem than it is elsewhere in the world. This can also impair the functioning of the Spleen and Stomach, leading to problems of sour belching, nausea and abdominal distention.

Chinese dietary theories are highly developed and will not receive more than a passing mention here. Different foods are thought to have different energies (hot, cold, sweet, greasy) which if eaten in excess can harm the functions of different organs. To cite one example, the Spleen likes dryness and warmth and over-consumption of cold energy foods (cold drinks, raw fruits and vegetables) can harm the Spleen Yang and cause diarrhea and abdominal pain.

Other factors that can influence someone's health include consumption of alcohol, tobacco and other drugs. Even vitamins and minerals, if taken incorrectly, can do more harm than good.

PHYSICAL ACTIVITY

To be healthy, it is important to balance exercise and rest in daily life. Regular exercise can harmonize the circulation of Qi and Blood. Movements in Tai Chi and Qi Gong are especially helpful. But excessive exercise or physical overwork can deplete Spleen Qi, leading to Qi and Blood Deficiencies, or if heavy lifting is involved the Kidneys can be weakened. And overuse of a particular part of the body through repetitive motion can lead to Qi stagnation in that area.

In Chinese medical texts, excessive sexual activity is considered a separate cause of disease. Male ejaculation is thought to deplete

Kidney Essence and reduce one's overall vitality. Some classics even provide guidelines for frequency of ejaculation. For women, multiple childbirths spaced too closely together can deplete Blood and weaken the Kidneys.

SCARS AND TRAUMA

Scars and traumatic injuries can interrupt the flow of Qi, especially when they cross an acupuncture channel. As will be explained in Chapters 10 and 11, such an interruption can lead to serious problems, even to cancer, later in life.

IMPROPER MEDICAL TREATMENT

In both Western and Oriental Medicines, incorrect treatments can be performed. Unnecessary surgeries and improper medications can do more harm than good. People even get surgery that they don't need, and any surgical intrusion into the body can disrupt Qi circulation. But an inaccurate herbal prescription can also be damaging to someone's health, and an acupuncture treatment applied by rote without taking a patient's unique condition into account may not be very effective.

IMPROPER QI GONG PRACTICE

Qi Gong has become more widely known and practiced over the past few years. However, there are now so many books and instructors that it is possible to get incorrect or incomplete information. People have made themselves sicker by moving or breathing in the wrong fashion. I will explain how this can happen in my next book, which will present my own Qi Gong practice.

ASTRONOMICAL INFLUENCES

The Chinese classics outline how Qi flows through the 12 Channels during every 24-hour period. Similarly, Qi ebbs and flows over the course of a month. This appears to follow the moon's gravitational pull like the tides in the ocean or people's moods. Sunspots which disturb radio waves also affect the flow of Qi in the body.

TECHNOLOGICAL INFLUENCES

Twentieth Century humans are affected by many factors that the authors of the classics did not have to address. The air and water have become polluted with toxic substances. Everywhere we go it is noisy. People are constantly bombarded by electromagnetic fields from high voltage wires and generators, and by radiation from television sets, computers, and microwave ovens. Injuries can come from tools and machinery that did not exist when the classics of medicine were written, and victims of violence or warfare are today wounded by bullets and explosives rather than arrows and spears.

These days, everyone sits and rides in cars or takes public transportation instead of walking, which is bad enough for one's health, even without the possibility of getting into accidents that hurt backs and necks. These injuries are painful by themselves and can impair the circulation of Qi and Blood through the acupuncture channels.

Infection

There are of course many pathogens that can make you sick, including bacteria, viruses, fungus, parasites, and insects. The Chinese did not develop the idea of germ theory until Ye Tien Si, who wrote about 1200 A.D. during the Song Dynasty. He was the first to present the idea that specific pathogens caused specific diseases.

Spirit Possession[22]

Modern medicine, whether in Asia or the West, rejects the idea that a spirit or devil can make you sick. But many cultures have believed that someone can be possessed. If you practice fasting Qi Gong meditation for longer than three weeks, you can begin to sense whether someone else is possessed by a spirit or devil. If someone needs exorcism by acupuncture, I can recommend a relative in China who is an expert. This is serious business and not to be fooled with.

Genetics

Many conditions are inherited from one's parents. Weak organs, physical malformations, mental retardation, and many diseases can all be genetically related. This is similar to the idea of Essence in Chinese medicine, in which a person's Essence is formed at conception out of the Essences of the parents.

STRESS

We are living in a stressful age. But it is really nothing new. Hans Selye, a professor at Montreal University, introduced "Stress Theory" in 1938, but later confessed that he had gotten the idea from a Latin translation of *The Yellow Emperor's Internal Medicine* (Nei Jing) written over 2,000 years ago.

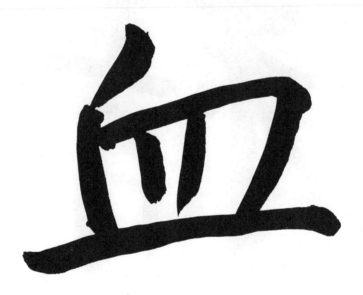

XUE(BLOOD)

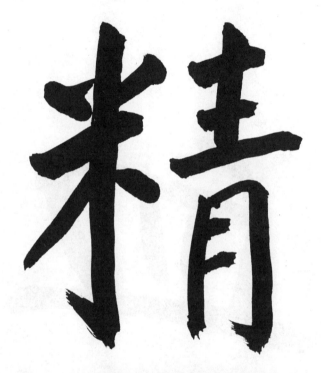

JING(ESSENCE)

Chapter 5

History of Oriental Medicine

In the early 1970s, some doctors of Chinese medicine visited the United States and hypothesized about the origins of acupuncture in an interview in *The New York Times*. They suggested that in ancient times warriors came back from the battle field with a variety of arrow, spear, and sword wounds. It was observed that wounds in particular parts of the body seemed to somehow cure diseases unrelated to the wounds. Out of these discoveries, more experiments were done leading to the discovery of acupuncture points.

This sounds like a logical explanation. It even includes Western-style scientific experimentation in the development of acupuncture. But it does not take into account the nature of Qi flow in the human body. Injuries or wounds occurring at any acupuncture point or crossing a channel will disturb the flow of Qi and be much more likely to cause problems than to stimulate the flow of Qi at the point of the wound.

A much more imaginative explanation takes off from a common theme in Asian fairy tales. An old man wearing a white robe and a long white beard appears to another man, usually in the mountains, and gives him a book before disappearing into the mist. Sometimes it is a martial arts book, sometimes a book on medicine. Some people say that this old man is actually an extraterrestrial bringing knowledge to the human race from the stars. These days, of course, many people in the West believe they have been contacted by UFOs, so perhaps this does not seem to be an outrageous idea to them. But I think it is more likely that what appeared was the spirit of a dead Taoist who had lived for many years in the mountains.

It is safe to say that the origins of acupuncture and Oriental Medicine go far back into history and that no one has the definitive answers. As you will see, much still waits for more research, and at least in China the founders of medicine are more mythic than historic. Some historians have described China as a giant marketplace to which people traveled from all over the known world and displayed their arts and culture to the Chinese, who recorded what they saw and incorporated parts into their own culture.

CHINA

In approximately 3000 B.C.E., the legendary figure Fu Xi is said to have lived in China. He is credited with developing the Ba Gua (Eight Trigrams) and writing the *I Ching*[23]. He is also referred to as the inventor of writing, musical instruments, fishing, and many other Chinese cultural arts.

Shen Nong, the father of Chinese herbal medicine, lived around 2800 B.C.E. He is said to have tasted seventy different substances every day as he established the art of medicine. His pharmacopoeia (Shen Nong Ben Cao Jing) contained 365 different herbs, 240 of which were plants and the remainder minerals, insects and other animal parts.

Much of the early history of Chinese medicine has been lost or destroyed. It is believed that a hospital was established during the Zhou Dynasty in 722 B.C.E. where acupuncture was used and that medical texts, and even the earliest licensing exams, date from this time. Unfortunately, between 221-206 B.C.E., during the Qin Dynasty from which China takes its name, Emperor Shih Hwang both built the Great Wall and burnt all the books, including those dealing with medicine. Although surely some books survived the destruction, nothing predating this time is known to exist today. The oldest books in China, which include medical books and the *Tao Te Ching*, are the silk manuscripts that were discovered in Ma Huang Tui in 1973 and date back to around 200 A.D. Another trove of important historical books was revealed to the outside world in 1850 by a monk who was keeping them in a cave along the Silk Road in Dun Huang in northwest China.

Sometime between 200 and 100 B.C.E., the *Huang Ti Nei Jing* or *Yellow Emperor's Internal Medicine* was written, supposedly by the Yellow Emperor himself. (Actually, any Chinese emperor in this period was called Huang Ti. Huang means yellow and refers to the gold color which was considered favorable for the Emperor's robes.) The book itself is structured as a series of conversations between the Yellow Emperor and his minister, Chi Bo. It is divided into two parts, the Su Wen or "Plain Questions" and the Ling Shu or "Spiritual Pivot." Some of the topics that are covered include Five Element Theory, Yin/Yang Theory, Acupuncture Theory, and the effects of weather and disease. Throughout Chinese history many books have been written as commentaries on the *Huang Ti Nei Jing* and it is still considered a fundamental classic of Chinese medicine today.

During the same era, Lao Tzu[24] wrote the *Tao Te Ching*.[25] As with the Yellow Emperor, Lao Tzu may not be an historical figure, but this work is still the foundation of Taoism. Later, in 25 B.C.E., another Taoist classic, *Tai Ping Jing*, appeared. It discussed the circulation of Qi and Blood, acupuncture, and the idea that illness arose from sin. Recipes for longevity are also given. Zhang Tao Ling described the effects of charms, incantations and magic in 74 A.D. Prayer was considered one of the thirteen branches of medicine.

Around 25 A.D., the *Nan Jing*, or *Classic on Difficulty*, was written. It is attributed to Qin Yueren, who was said to have been an innkeeper who learned medicine from a wandering physician who was his guest. The *Nan Jing* emphasized pulse diagnosis and needle manipulation and contains the earliest discussion of the extraordinary meridians. It has been especially influential in the development of acupuncture in Japan.

Buddhism[26] arrived in China around 67 A.D. from India. With it came the ancient tradition of Ayurvedic Medicine[27], which influenced Chinese medicine as the Indian philosophy of the Bhagavad Gita[28] had earlier influenced the *Tao Te Ching*.

In 169 A.D., Zhang Zhong Jing was the mayor of Changsha, a city in the northern part of China. There were epidemics occurring in the city, and he wrote "Essay on Typhoid" and *Shang Han Lun* or *Treatise on Cold Induced Diseases*. Thanks to the efforts of Wang Shu Ho, who edited his work in the third century, many herbal prescriptions have been saved that are still in use today. Zhang Zhong Jing's work is also important for his emphasis on differential diagnosis as the foundation for a treatment plan.

The famous Buddhist monk Bodhidharma arrived at the Shaolin Temple from India in 527 A.D. and was appalled to discover that the monks there were in such poor health from their hours of motionless meditation that they were unable to stay awake. He introduced exercises to strengthen their bodies which over the centuries have evolved into many of the Chinese martial arts. This style of Buddhism also strongly influenced Zen in Japan.

During the Sui Dynasty (589-618 A.D.), a decree was issued that four categories of people could administer acupuncture and herbs. They were dietitians, physicians, surgeons, and veterinarians. By this time, farmers had taken up the cultivation of many medicinal herbs rather than gathering everything in the wild.

In the Tang Dynasty, these categories were further refined and four more categories were added to the Sui Dynasty list: pediatricians, specialists in adult diseases, what we would today call otolaryngologists (eye, ear, nose, mouth, teeth, and throat specialists), and practitioners of massage and cupping[29]. Doctors were divided into four categories: physicians, acupuncturists, masseurs, and exorcists. (Superstition and the use of magic was on the increase during the Tang Dynasty.) The medical profession was not held in high esteem by the mainstream Confucianists of the period, but was supported by the Imperial court, which sponsored the Imperial Medical College. The College in turn provided exclusive health care to the royal family until the end of the Qing Dynasty and the establishment of the Republic of China under Sun Yat Sen.

During the Song Dynasty (960-1279 A.D.) the first formal medical school was established and licensing exams for doctors were instituted. Prior to this time, medical training consisted of apprenticeships, generally either father to son or master to disciple.

In the twelfth century, Ye Tien Si wrote *Wen Bing Lun*, which examined the effects of heat and warm weather inducing disease. He lived near the Yangtze River in southern China. In this climate, severe infections spread quickly and could prove toxic. They were difficult to treat using the strategies of Zhang Zhong Jing. Instead, Ye observed how exposure to different pathogens caused specific epidemic diseases, anticipating germ theory in the West. He formulated new herbal prescriptions to counter febrile diseases, and these formulas are still widely used.

In 1796 the English physician Edward Jenner developed a vaccine for smallpox, a major step forward in Western medicine. Yet one thousand years earlier, practitioners in China and Tibet collected pus from smallpox lesions and blew it through a straw into people's noses to help them develop immunity to the disease. I suspect that this similar discovery followed very different paths in Asia and the West. Western people believe that civilization has developed through the use of logic and reason and that technological advances are the result of applications of the scientific method. But in Asia, intuition and insight are thought to play much greater roles. Many advances in Oriental Medicine have resulted from periods of fasting meditation; intuitive, spontaneous knowledge acquired and refined through internal Yin training and practices. Yet it is interesting that these drastically different approaches can at times lead to the same result.

Chinese medicine continued to develop over the centuries completely isolated from the developments in science taking place in the West. Because of this, it was viewed by many Twentieth Century modernizers as an impediment to the development of a scientific medical system in China. Things deteriorated so far that the Health Ministry declared Chinese medicine and the use of acupuncture illegal in 1929. However this decision was unpopular and many people continued to seek out traditional practitioners. Mao Zedong and the Communist government permitted controlled use of traditional Chinese medicine even during the 1930s in Yenan. In 1950, schools and hospitals were opened that taught both Chinese and Western medicines, a situation that has continued ever since. Today in China there are five-year programs in Traditional Chinese Medicine (TCM) and Western medicine, and students in the latter also learn some TCM as part of their education. Graduates must pass licensing exams before they are allowed to practice.

INDIA

The Ayurvedic system of medicine has been practiced in India since 4000 B.C.E. Although a very different approach, the Ayurvedic system uses many of the same diagnostic tools and treatments that Chinese medicine does. The tongue and pulse are checked and urine samples are examined. Herbs are used as medicinal substances and practices like yoga and meditation recommended for health purposes. Even Five Element Theory shows strong similarities to Ayurvedic tastes and the influences of the organs are the same. Today there are colleges of Ayurvedic Medicine in India just as there are TCM colleges in China.

Probably as Buddhism traveled along the trade routes between India and China, medical information did as well. There does appear to have been a good deal of cultural exchange. In his recent translation of the *Tao Te Ching*, the first based on the ancient Ma Huang Tui silk manuscripts, Walter Mair includes an appendix which describes a close relationship between the foundation of Taoism and the Bhagavad Gita, the masterwork of Hindu scripture.

The Chinese have always claimed that the legendary Fu Xi wrote the *I Ching* around 3000 B.C.E. But the oldest existing depiction of the Eight Trigram symbol was found not in China, but in the jungles of India. Perhaps Fu Xi was from India himself, or brought back Yin/Yang theory and its symbol from his travels there.

Much later, after the Islamic invasion of India in 1192 A.D. and the establishment of the Sultanate of Delhi, the Muslim armies destroyed many Buddhist temples, and thousands of monks fled to Nepal and Tibet. Some of these monks later made their way to China, probably carrying Indian cultural practices and medical information with them.

In any case, it is clear that India and China have influenced each other throughout their long histories, even if the Chinese do prefer to portray themselves as having developed their culture without much interaction with other peoples.

KOREA

Chinese medicine was being practiced in Korea during the Han Dynasty in China in 206 B.C.E. It may be even older than this, although no records have been found. Korean attitudes towards medicine were influenced by the Chinese Confucian tradition, which did not hold doctors in high esteem. As a result, medicine was practiced by the middle class rather than the aristocracy. Medical training was passed down from father to son or master to apprentice. For at least one thousand years prior to the Japanese occupation in 1910, during the Koryo and Chosun Kingdoms, there was a competitive examination for the post of Imperial Court Physician. After Korea regained its independence from the Japanese in 1945, the remaining doctors of the Imperial Court established a school for Oriental Medicine which is now a six year college in Seoul. Today there are many universities teaching Oriental Medicine in Korea, and graduates must pass a licensing examination before they are allowed to practice.

JAPAN

Japan was first introduced to Chinese medicine by visiting Koreans during the Three Kingdoms period (37 B.C.E.-668 A.D.). Direct contacts between Chinese and Japanese physicians began during the Tang Dynasty (619-907 A.D.). Over the centuries, the Japanese have developed their own unique approaches to the practice of Oriental Medicine.

Over the last 200 years, the blind were specially trained in acupuncture and massage. They have developed highly refined palpatory approaches to diagnosis using their enhanced tactile sensitivity. One blind acupuncturist, Sugiyama Waichi, revolutionized the practice of acupuncture in the early 1800s by inventing the insertion tube. The tube makes it possible to insert even very fine needles easily into the patient, making acupuncture a less painful experience. He later became the Shogun's acupuncturist and was granted the official title Sugiyama Ken Gyo, or teacher.

After the surrender of Japan to the United States in 1945, General Douglas MacArthur, the Supreme Commander of the Allied Powers, tried to ban acupuncture, just as Chiang Kai-shek had previously attempted to do in China. But MacArthur was no more successful than Chiang had been, as the different schools and practitioners of acupuncture in Japan set aside their differences and united in opposition to the attempt to outlaw their profession.

In the postwar period, Japan has been the site of many innovations in acupuncture. One of the most important figures has been Dr. Yoshio Manaka. Among his inventions has been the ion pumping cord, which connects needles in different acupuncture points by means of a wire and diode. The cord, which Dr. Manaka first used on wartime burn victims, circulates the body's own Qi externally to facilitate treatment.

The system of training is rather different in Japan than it is elsewhere in Asia. There are separate five-year colleges that teach acupuncture, moxibustion, and herbal medicine, and separate licenses for each treatment modality. As a result, practitioners tend to specialize more narrowly than elsewhere.

Many different Asian peoples have made important contributions to the development of the art of healing. Sometimes this perspective is lost as different countries try to claim credit for themselves by ignoring the contributions of others. For example, Five Element Style acupuncture theory was formulated by the Korean priest Sa Am Do In about 400 years ago. Yet in China and Japan as well as Europe and America, where his approach is widely used, his name is never mentioned. It is only in Korea that he is credited with being a major acupuncture innovator.

Ear acupuncture is widely practiced in China today, yet Chinese textbooks and charts of ear points do not credit Dr. Paul Nogier, the French neurosurgeon who, 20 years ago, discovered 80% of the ear points currently in use. Historically the Chinese only employed a few points and ear acupuncture did not form a comprehensive system prior to Dr. Nogier's research.

I believe that it is best to share the credit. The basic fundamental theory of Yin/Yang probably came to China from India, as did the Buddhist meditation techniques called Chan in China and Zen in Japan. Some people believe that even Qi Gong and Tai Chi came originally from India and Tibet. So when I am asked about the medicine I practice, I choose to describe it as Oriental Medicine rather than Chinese or Korean.

Chapter 6
Yin/Yang Theory

The Chinese characters for Yin/Yang refer to the shady and sunny sides of a hill, respectively. Over the course of the day, the amount of sun and shade on the hill changes as the sun moves across the sky. Similarly, Yin and Yang are always in motion.

Yin/Yang theory has its origins in the dualist philosophy of ancient India. The term Sanskrit term Hata, as in Hata Yoga, has a similar meaning to Yin and Yang in Chinese. In India, it was thought that God and the Devil possessed equal abilities and co-existed in the world just as other dualities like day and night, man and woman, Heaven and Earth did.

The *I Ching*, one of the oldest texts in existence, was written in China about 4,000 years ago. It explains the principles of change. The *I Ching* argues that there are three kinds of changes occurring in the universe. In the first type, the universe seems to be constantly changing in a complicated manner, yet paradoxically the principles of change are very simple. With the second kind of change, the universe appears static even though it is actually changing by Yin/Yang principles. Finally, in the third type of change, the universe reveals that the only unchangeable principle is the principle of change itself.

Yin qualities include soft, cold, fluid-like and slow activity, even motionless, night, woman, the Moon, the Earth. Yang qualities include hard, hot, solid, active like the day, man, the Sun and Heaven. The comparative adjectives that describe the phenomena of the universe sound like Yin and Yang dualities: big and small, wide and narrow, hot and cold, strong and weak, bright and dark. In describing the universe, these adjectives do not employ absolute concepts. Instead they emphasize the relativity of phenomena.

Any phenomenon that has existed as predominantly Yang for a long period of time must necessarily become Yin at some point, and vice versa. In human history we see that a nation's power and prosperity never lasts forever at its apogee. And in an individual's life, health, fame, and fortune constantly change instead of remaining at a peak.

When Western people see the Yin/Yang symbol they sometimes think of it as day and night, as a representation of the pro and con of Western logic, as black and white, or as polar opposites as my theory indicates (figure 6-1). But there is no Yin/Yang symbol like this as there would be if it represented a stationary concept like Western logic.

These types of lines are often seen in modern mathematics and the stock market. They represent constant change and make up the original Yin/Yang symbol.

I think of Yin/Yang as not only day and night but also as sunset and dawn, the transitional moving stages between the opposite poles. When you are diagnosing a patient, you must not only correctly identify the nature of the disease (Hot or Cold, Damp or Dry, Yin or Yang) but also in which way it is progressing (see Figure 6-2).

This fish-shaped Yin/Yang sign symbolizes the seed of Yang within Yin and Yin within Yang. Sensibility and softness are often found within strong men, and strong will power and physical energy in fragile women(see Figure 6-3).

This triple color shape is found only in Korean and Tibetan cultures. The symbol appears on small drums that are played by women in both countries. It is also seen as a design on Korean fans and on the gates of old traditional Korean houses. The three primary colors are used in this design. Red symbolizes Heaven and Blue the Earth as in other Yin/Yang symbols, but here the Yellow is added to represent humanity (see Figure 6-4).

Korea and Tibet have other connections to each other. Traditional costumes are similar, in particular the dress worn by the shamans. The phenotype[30] of the Korean people is similar to that of the Mongols, but their genotype[31] is closer to that of Central Asians like the Tibetans. I like to think that my affinity for and understanding of Yin/Yang theory is in part due to DNA in the nuclei of every cell in my body that has been passed down to me from Tibetan masters of antiquity.

Recently the Japanese have applied Yin/Yang principles to the mechanical workings of their subway system. It stops and starts gradually, flowing smoothly without any abrupt motion. In these modern times, the use of computers seems to make peoples' thinking increasingly rigid like computer logic: yes/no, on/off, and so on. I think that modern people should add Yin/Yang theory to their mental repertoire for the sake of increasing flexibility of mind.

One of the first and most difficult things facing Korean students when they arrive in America is a one-hour essay in the form of a questionnaire. They have problems with this because of their cultural upbringing. Western philosophy tries to explain everything in terms of absolutes like yes or no, pro or con. This is quite different from Oriental philosophy, which explains things in terms of relativity or Yin/Yang. Even though Korean students use correct syntax and grammar when they are writing answers for the essay/questionnaire, they are often assumed to lack logical cohesion because the Western way assumes a clear cut yes or no for an answer.

I find that most Koreans use Yin/Yang theory unconsciously. They compare the two sides of any question and then come up with a conclusion relevant to the present moment. This way of thinking is prominent in the editorials of Korean newspapers and in the daily conversations of Korean people. Once, at a meeting for the unification of North and South Korea, I heard one person say to another, "Don't talk in terms of pro and con." To me, this comment reflects this unconscious use of Yin/Yang theory. I think that because we Koreans use Yin/Yang theory in our daily lives like this, we can come to some agreement to co-exist, both sides yielding to understand the other's strengths and weaknesses. If this can be done in any small way, this could be the first step towards the unification of North and South Korea.

In my opinion, trying to find an absolute set of values may be good for the natural sciences, but with people in the social sciences flexibility of thinking and the acceptance of Yin/Yang theory seem to be of great value in trying to understand the world as it is today.

Korean elders like to use traditional proverbs that say "Yin land will become Yang land and Yang land will become Yin land," "A mouse hole could get sunshine one day," "A flower blossom will

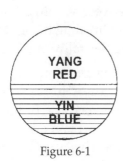

Figure 6-1

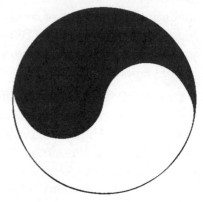

Figure 6-2

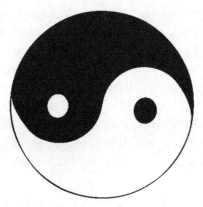

Figure 6-3

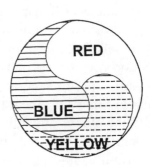

Figure 6-4

last only ten days, the full moon will wane. Prosperity and failure are the inevitable course of life."

The famous Chinese war novel *The Three Kingdoms Warfare* begins by stating that in relationships between countries in this world, if nations have been united for a long time, separation becomes inevitable. If they have been separated for a long time, unification becomes inevitable. When one tries to understand classical Chinese fiction or poetry, either at the level of an individual paragraph or stanza or an entire work, one should look for the contrasting verse, sentence, plot, or character.

Near the end of the movie The Godfather Part I, scenes of a baby being baptized in a church and two rival Mafia gangs shooting it out with machine guns are alternated quickly to create an impression of life and death, war and peace, the Yin and Yang of human tragedy. In The Godfather Part II, a small Sicilian boy landed at Ellis Island in New York Harbor. He was sick, weak and could not speak a word of English. He grew up to become the Mafia Godfather. This Yin/Yang formula is the opposite of Shakespearean tragedy, where people from the aristocratic class have their lives and positions ruined.

In the personals columns of newspapers like the *Boston Globe*, people run advertisements searching for lovers and potential spouses. These ads are divided into sections in which men seek women, women seek men, men seek men, and women seek women. I have yet to see sections specifically for bisexual men or women seeking each other. This variety illustrates the fact that although the sexual types of our physical bodies are either male or female, sexual preferences are much more complex, just as Yin/Yang theory is much more nuanced and complex than simple dualism.

The following observations show how to use Yin/Yang theory to analyze individuals physically and psychologically in order to develop a diagnosis and treatment plan.

MUSICIANS

Guitar Player - Dress and attitude unsettled. Moves a lot. Usually single: Yang type.

Pianist - More settled in dress and attitude. Keeps still. Usually

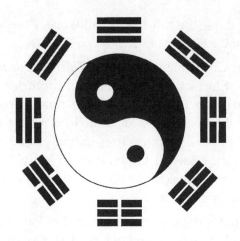

Figure 6-5

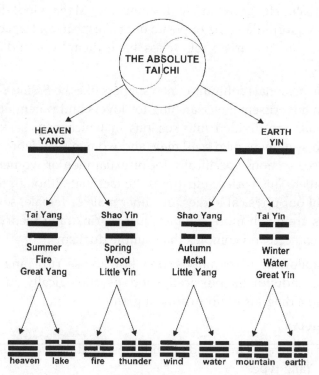

Figure 6-6

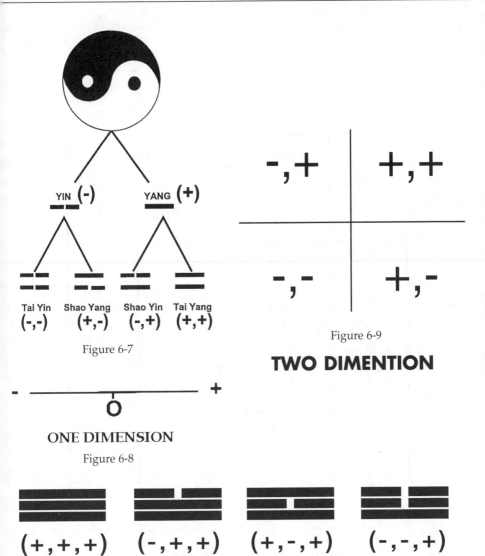

YIN (-)   **YANG (+)**

Tai Yin   Shao Yang   Shao Yin   Tai Yang
(-,-)   (+,-)   (-,+)   (+,+)

Figure 6-7

-,+   +,+

-,-   +,-

Figure 6-9

TWO DIMENTION

-            +
           O

ONE DIMENSION

Figure 6-8

(+,+,+)   (-,+,+)   (+,-,+)   (-,-,+)

(+,+,-)   (-,+,-)   (+,-,-)   (-,-,-)

THREE DIMENSION

Figure 6-10

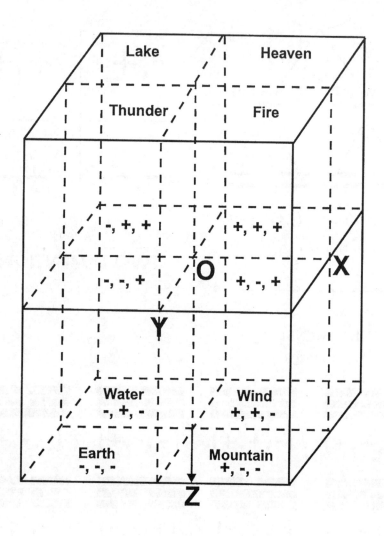

THREE DIMENSION

Figure 6-11

married: Yin type.

We can of course divide guitar players and pianists themselves, just as Yin and Yang can be further subdivided into Yin or Yang within Yin, etc. A folk guitar player who constantly travels around the country with only his wooden guitar demonstrates different characteristics than a rock musician with tons of electronic equipment who requires assistants and heavy transportation to go on the road. Without support the musician is forced to be as sedentary as any farmer.

AUTOMOBILE RACER

This is a very dangerous sport, very masculine in character and involving wild action and risk of death. Therefore we would expect that a race car driver will be a masculine, strong-looking individual. On the contrary, however, they are usually relatively small. Perhaps they are trying to overcome their small stature and physical inferiority complex and prove their strength by mastering powerful machinery.

I have found that in general a one-armed person is extremely Yang and more active than a person with both arms. A one-legged person, conversely, is much more Yin; less active and more of a thinker. A classic example is Talleyrand, the lamed French Foreign Minister who first aided Napoleon and later helped to destroy him and restore the monarchy in France and the autocratic status quo throughout Europe. Another would be Louis Pasteur, the nineteenth century French chemist who made crucial discoveries in immunology and microbiology.

A person with an outgoing personality tends to talk about problems with friends, relatives or a therapist. This way he does not keep worries and anger inside but instead can get advice and feel better. An introspective person, however, tends to keep problems inside. This can potentially lead to stomach ulcers and even the development of cancer.

Parents are always advising their children in terms of Yin/Yang balance whether they are aware they are doing so or not.

"Why do you spend all your time playing outside? You need to read more books and study instead."

"Why do you sit in front of the computer all day? I want you to go out and play like the other kids."

Parents always want their children's mental and physical activities to be in balance.

Earlier I described some of the qualities of Yin/Yang interaction. These can be summarized as four principles:

Everything contains the opposite qualities of Yin and Yang.

- Yin and Yang exist in interdependence.
- Yin and Yang balance and control each other.
- Yin and Yang change into each other.

In order to illustrate these principles, examine the development of Chinese philosophy before and during the Warring States Period (403-221 B.C.E.). This was a period of great turmoil following the collapse of the Zhou Dynasty during which there was no central authority. Prior to this, three philosophical schools developed, all of which focused on the external and objective source of ethics. Confucius (551-479 B.C.E.) stressed manner, etiquette, and formality in a strongly enforced social hierarchy in order to keep the peace. Lao Tzu (ca. 570 B.C.E.) and his Taoist successors rejected the status quo as exemplified by Confucius, stating that governments, rulers, and kings were not necessary to achieve or maintain harmony in the land. Instead, emphasis was placed on serene contemplation as the source of personal growth and the way to peace. Mu Ga (480-390 B.C.E.) also rejected Confucianism's rigid etiquette and formality, placing more emphasis on the practical and economic side of life, advocating equality and love for each other.

Mencius (372-289 B.C.E.), one of Confucius' successors, propounded a theory of good nature. It was his belief that man is born generally good-natured with an innate sense of etiquette, virtue, and righteousness. However, these qualities did not guarantee that an individual's life would develop in a virtuous direction. Being surrounded by bad circumstances during life could change virtue to evil and what might be a virtue under certain circumstances, become evil in other situations. To develop virtue would require proper training and cultivation.

Following Mencius, Confucianism emphasized the internal and

subjective views of morality that he had developed. However Sun-Tzu (320-225 B.C.E) rearranged Confucianism by emphasizing an essentially negative or bad nature theory of life. He denied the authority of Heaven, which he described as the sky rather than as a source of ethical standards, as Confucius and Mencius had stated. This separation of man from Heaven required a new set of ethics for the protection of the individual. Sun-Tzu asserted that these ethics were universal and would help to rein in people's dangerous desires. However, these rules could only be applied according to each man's ability and social class. Despite this loophole, Sun-Tzu's view that human nature was intrinsically evil never gained wide popularity.

Western students of Oriental Medicine or martial arts often feel that they are faced with contradictory theories and struggle to determine which idea is correct and which is wrong, which teacher is telling the truth and which is passing on incorrect or false teachings. But there will always be problems when you try to judge Oriental theories with Western linear logic. Yin/Yang theory, however, makes room for the coexistence of equally valid contradictory theories.

According to legend, the *I Ching* was written ca. 2100 B.C.E by the Emperor Fu-Hsi. Fu-Hsi was believed to be a sage who studied the patterns of Nature, including those of the Heavens, the Earth, the animals, the seasons, his own body, and both fire and water before completing his book. Throughout history there have been many opinions on the true author of this book, but it is agreed that the *I Ching* is the origin of medical philosophy. It was even praised by Confucius as making use of the patterns of the Universe to shed light on the patterns of human affairs, especially as related to medicine. However, Confucius also stated that the *I Ching* was so complex that after a lifetime of study he did not feel that he had completely comprehended it. Its complexity has allowed it to serve as a source of inspiration to many political, scientific, and medical theories. Within the past fifty years, some scholars have tried to apply modern scientific formulas and mathematics to a study of the *I Ching*. This has been of interest to me and I would like to introduce my personal theory relating mathematics to the *I Ching*.

I have found that even though the Chinese believe that they were the originators of the Yin/Yang symbol, Indian philosophy is responsible for the original idea. Indian Buddhism's philosophical view divides this universe into three dimensions: Front/Back, Left/Right, and Above/Below. Even when they pray, their objectives are more than three dimensional as compared to, say, the Christian ceremony.

During the morning and evening prayers in a Buddhist temple, four distinct sounds are created to make four different requests. Bells are used to send Buddha's message to any of the dead who are suffering in Hell. Drums ask for the salvation of all living things on the earth at that moment. Thin sheets of metal are beaten to guide lost spirits in the atmosphere up to Heaven. A wooden fish is struck like a gong, to send Buddha's protection to anything living under the water. Hence the four sounds, the four types of prayer call for the guidance and protection of all creatures on Earth or in the sea and of all lost or suffering souls of the dead.

I have also found that the symbols used for Yin and Yang in the *I Ching* (A broken line [- -] for Yin and a solid line [__] for Yang) match exactly with the "-" and "+" symbols used in the modern Cartesian coordinate system. When combined to form trigrams they resemble the bar codes that are read by cash registers today.

The *I Ching* is based on the foundation of the eight trigrams, the "ba kua" or "pal gue." These eight trigrams can be seen as a three dimensional Cartesian entity. Similarly, the human body can be described in this way. Let "X" represent Left or Right, "Y" represent Front or Back, "Z" represent Above or Below, and "O" represent the center. These coordinates can be used to determine any position on someone's body.

For the last four thousand years, the Chinese have thought that Tai Yang, Shao Yang, Tai Yin, and Shao Yin corresponded to the four seasons or the four primary directions. Their interpretation of the eight trigrams was also two dimensional, adding Northeast, Northwest, Southeast and Southwest to the four directions. However the images for the eight trigrams in the *I Ching* are three dimensional, such as mountain, lake, or heaven. These geographical features associated with the trigrams connect the spatial outlooks of the Eastern Yin/Yang and the Western Cartesian coordinate systems. However it must be emphasized that unlike the rigid limits of the Western system, the boundaries of the trigram regions are both fluid and permeable and the regions themselves represent only predispositions, not rigid definitions (see Figures 6-5 through 6-11).

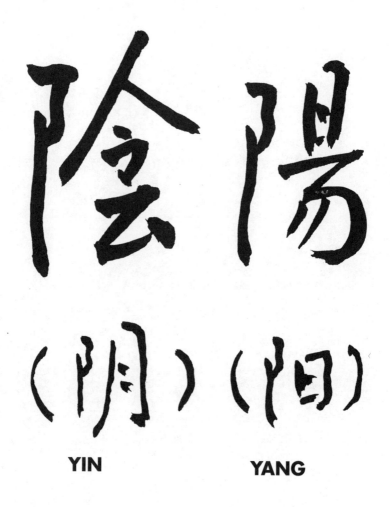

YIN   YANG

Chapter 7

Five Element Theory

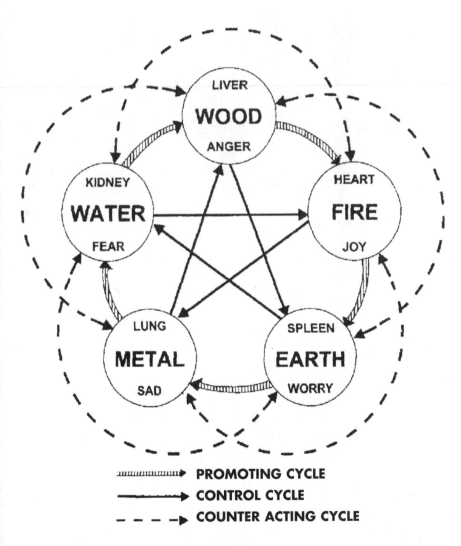

Figure 7-1

Five Element Theory Chart

Element	WOOD	FIRE	EARTH	METAL	WATER
Yin/Yang Organ	Liver/Gallbladder	Heart/Small Intestine	Spleen/Stomach	Lung/Large Intestine	Kidney/Urinary Bladder
Sense Organ	Eye	Tongue	Mouth	Nose	Ear
Tissue	Tendons	Blood	Muscle	Skin & Body Hair	Bone & Head Hair
Emotion	Anger	Joy	Excess Thought	Grief	Fear
Season	Spring	Summer	Mid-Summer	Autumn	Winter
Harmful Weather	Wind	Heat	Damp	Dryness	Cold
Development	Germination	Growth	Transformation	Harvest	Storage
Color	Green	Red	Yellow	White	Black
Flavor	Sour	Bitter	Sweet	Pungent	Salty
Direction	East	South	Center	West	North

Table 7-1

The ancient Chinese thought that this world was made up of wood, fire, earth, metal, and water. Everything in nature, including human disease, was believed to have been caused by interactions between these five elements. Figure 7-1 illustrates these interactions: the promoting and controlling cycles. The promoting cycle brings growth and development, for example water nourishes wood and enables it to grow. The controlling cycle, on the other hand, can prevent an element from growing, as wood can be cut down by metal.

The promoting cycle involves the following interactions. Wood burns to create fire, fire leaves ashes that become earth, earth is where metal is found, molten metal becomes water, and water nourishes wood and helps it grow.

The controlling cycle operates as follows: wood grows in soil and its roots can crack any earth, even rock. Fire can melt metal. Earth can be mounded up into a dam to control water. Metal can be made into an ax to chop wood. Water can extinguish fire.

These two cycles set up five possible interactions between organs that need to be considered when analyzing any organ problem. Let's take the Liver as an example of how this works.

1.   A Liver (Wood) problem may simply be due to a disharmony of the Liver itself.

2.   Liver can be affected by the Kidney (Water), the element before it on the promoting cycle. This is also described as "The mother affecting the son."

3.   A Liver problem can be caused by a weakened Heart (Fire), the element following it on the promoting cycle. This is called "The son affecting the mother."

4.   If a Liver problem is caused by a Lung (Metal) problem it is called "Metal over controlling Wood." Remember that Metal precedes Wood on the controlling cycle.

5.   A Liver problem can also be caused by an excess of Spleen (Earth), the element following it on the controlling cycle. This is "Earth counter-attacking Wood."

There are two main treatment principles employed in Five Element Theory. If an organ is underactive or deficient, as in the case of a chronic disease, the mother element is tonified. For example, if the Liver (Wood) is weak, the Kidney (Water) should be tonified. If an organ is overactive or excess, as in the case of an acute febrile disease, then the son should be sedated. In this case, if the Liver is overactive, then sedate the Heart (Fire).

The colors and tastes listed in the Five Element chart can be used for diagnostic purposes. For example, if a person comes into the office with a greenish complexion and a preference for sour flavors he or she could well have a Liver problem. Someone with a known Liver problem, a dark complexion and a preference for salty food probably has a Kidney problem that is affecting the Liver, or "The mother affecting her son."

Someone with a red complexion and bitter taste who begins to show a Liver problem could be said to have a Heart problem affecting the Liver, or "The son affecting his mother."

A patient with a Liver problem who begins to have digestive problems and a craving for sweet foods along with a green and yellow complexion would be described as "Wood controlling Earth," while someone with a Liver problem who began to demonstrate a Lung disharmony and a pale greenish complexion could be called "Metal counter-attacking Wood."

I find it interesting that the relationships between organs and tastes in Indian Ayurvedic Medicine are the same as the one described here for Chinese medicine. This is yet another example of the overlapping cross-influences between Indian and Chinese cultures that require much further study.

The *Neijing* describes how to control emotional problems using the controlling cycle of Five Element Theory. I have added some modern applications of this theory here.

Anger (Wood) can be controlled by sadness (Metal). A modern application of this idea suggests that since a patient with Liver problems is easily angered, this person should read sad novels and watch sad movies.

Joy (Fire) can be controlled by fear (Water). A patient with Heart problems often shows excessive joy or bounces easily up and down emotionally. This person should try watching scary movies or reading horror stories to control this. Excessive joy causes Qi to rise to the upper part of the body and the head, and horror movies can help bring the Qi back down to the lower part of the body. A person's Qi should be centered in the Dan Tien, an area located about one inch below the navel. It would make sense for movie producers to distribute horror films during the Summer, when the Heart is most active and people are most in need of something to draw their Qi back down.

Worry (Earth) can be controlled by anger (Wood). A patient with Spleen and Stomach problems tends to be pensive in nature and to worry too much about unimportant matters. This sort of person should watch political films and read about current affairs. The anger that is stimulated by much of what goes on in the world today can help to balance this over-worrying.

Sadness (Metal) can be controlled by joy (Fire). A patient with Lung problems is often sad. Such a person should be exposed to comedies and stories with happy endings to counteract this. When you say "Cheer up!" to someone who is sad you are actually applying Five Element Theory.

Fear (Water) can be controlled by over-thinking (Earth). Someone with Kidney problems is easily frightened. They should watch documentary or educational films or read about science to try to control this problem.

Women experience Premenstrual Syndrome (PMS) with a wide variety of symptoms. For some, physical pain is the biggest problem, while for others emotional difficulties are more pronounced. This variation can be understood by an application of Five Element Theory. If the patient has Liver (Wood) problems, they will display irritability and anger. If Heart (Fire), there will be excessive joy and/or anger. If Spleen (Earth), the patient will worry. If Lung (Metal), there will be sadness. Finally, if the patient has Kidney (Water) problems, fear will predominate.

Thousands of years ago as Chinese culture developed, paper was scarce and access was basically limited to the nobility. Because of this material scarcity and the complexity of written Chinese ideographs, long sentences were frequently shortened to four character verses. Therefore, when one reads Confucius, he says

"A wise man is like mountains.

A wise man is like water."

This is generally taken to mean that one kind of intellectual acts like mountains. They prefer a quiet place to study and meditate. But the other type of intellectual, people like businessmen, politicians, and military strategists, act like water with its variety of movements. This is the most widely agreed upon interpretation of this quotation amongst Confucian scholars. For me, however, Confucius is advising scholars to balance the

Yin and Yang aspects of their lives, to be like both mountains and water rather than one or the other. I think that this is pretty good advice and something that I have observed that many people in America do without even thinking about it. Many people who live near the ocean like to travel to the mountains, and people who dwell in the mountains often go to the beach for holidays.

How did Five Element Theory develop? The charts of correspondences have existed since antiquity, but they never come with information describing when, how, and where they were worked out. Were people surveyed? Did doctors keep records of all their patients? No one really knows. My favorite theory is that a Taoist master figured it all out during a period of fasting meditation and then just observed his patients and confirmed what had come to him in a moment of insight.

Everyone has noticed that during the heat of the Summer people are easily angered. This is the time of year when many mass murders take place and people go crazy with automatic weapons. Conversely, in the Winter when it is cold and gray, people become more depressed and many suicides take place.

Not long ago a 50 year-old woman with a pale, white complexion came to my office. She complained of a skin disease, psoriasis, around her elbow and knee. As I spoke with her, I learned that her mother died the previous Summer and that she was extremely sad. (She had come to my office in the Autumn, the dry season.) She also enjoyed eating pungent, hot spicy food. Finally, she suffered from bronchitis and pneumonia when she was eight years-old.

Much of what she displayed were symptoms associated with Metal. The time of year of her complaint, its dry nature, her preference for pungent foods, her early history of lung problems and her sadness all indicated a Metal disharmony. Therefore I advised her to avoid pungent spicy foods and trips to the West, especially during the Autumn. I also suggested that she should not read sad novels or television programs and to choose adventures or comedies instead.

Sometimes I like to think about applying Five Element Theory as a sort of variant on Darwinian evolutionary theory. According to Five Element Theory, people with Heart ailments should not visit or live in the southern regions of the U.S., especially during the heat of the Summer. Similarly, people with Kidney problems should not travel to the northern U.S. during the Winter. Probably people who live in the tropics have stronger hearts and people living in the Arctic have stronger kidneys. This is because over the generations people living in particular climatic zones have been genetically selected for traits, such as stronger hearts or kidneys, that give them a better chance of survival and reproduction. Of course, with the ease of movement in the modern world, it is easy for people to end up in regions for which their constitutions are poorly adapted, and health problems may result.

It should be remembered that Five Element Theory was conceived by the Chinese in accordance with their particular geographic surroundings and the types of weather found in different regions of their country. Since the United States has a similar geographic location in the Northern hemisphere, some of the concepts of Five Element Theory can be applied to the treatment of patients in North America. But to treat patients in the Southern Hemisphere the theory would have to be modified to take into account the reversed polar/equatorial orientation. For example, according to the theory, a patient with kidney disease should not go north in the Winter because of the colder temperatures found there. So in a country like Australia, a patient should be told to avoid the South and to move closer to the Equator.

There are many other parts of the world where these correspondences do not work very well at all. Take Russia as an example. It is certainly cold in the North, but much of southern Russia is awfully cold as well. Is it damper in the center of the country than elsewhere? Not as far as I know. And certainly it is not dry in the West at all.

Five Element Theory also states that a patient with lung disease should not travel to the West in the Autumn. This is because the air in Western China is very dry and contains pollen and dust that can easily cause allergic reactions, lung disease, and skin problems. Excessive sadness, the emotion of the Lungs, could also be triggered by this climate. This prohibition on travel to the West would also apply to the United States, where much of the Western regions are similarly dry.

I remember reading an article which gave an interesting Western medical perspective on this. In the Desert Southwest of the United States, there is a fungus called Coccidioidomycosis. It is found on dried animal feces and can be carried by the wind into the nostrils and then penetrates the lungs. It causes both skin diseases and lung problems in humans. Between 60-80% of local people test positively for exposure to this fungus without side effects. But if non-native people with lung problems spend a year in this part of the country, more than 80% of them will contact severe pneumonia, one-third will end up with permanent lung disease and a few will even die.

These climatic/directional correspondences would be meaningless, however, in island countries like England or Japan, or peninsular nations like Korea, Italy, or Greece, where there is less climatic variance between East and West. So it is important to consider climate and geography when applying Five Element Theory so that it does not degenerate into mere superstition.

People from cold climates, like the Eskimos, often suffer from severe dermatitis if they travel down to a warm climate during the summer. People from Tibet who find themselves living at a lower altitude with a warmer climate often have seriously high blood pressure, with a systolic pressure up around 300. In the Himalayas they have developed blood with an extraordinarily large number of red blood cells to conserve oxygen. Because of this, their blood density is higher than people living at lower altitudes, and if a Tibetan moves down to sea level the high density will cause higher than normal blood pressure. It will be difficult for them to reduce this unless they are able to practice Qi Gong for many hours a day like the Taoist masters in the old legends. Neither thirst, hunger, heat, nor cold could interfere with their body functions. But if this is not possible I would recommend that Tibetans try to live in areas as similar in terms of climate and altitude as possible.

Studies have shown that Korean emigrants to the U.S. and black men over forty years of age living in the northern U.S. have the highest incidences of stomach cancer of any ethnic groups in the country. I think that the Koreans are suffering from business stress while probably the black men are also suffering from stress caused by socio-economic problems that are not included in Five Element Theory.

Color interpretation is another area in which Five Element Theory is often misapplied. Some people have gone so far as to say that someone with a Liver problem has a preference for wearing green clothes in the springtime or that someone with a Heart problem would wear red in the Summer and so forth. I have not noticed too many patients with this dress color/disease correlation, except maybe people on St. Patrick's Day[32], who seem to like to wear green and drink too much, which can certainly damage their livers. It is true that St. Patrick's Day occurs at the beginning of spring and that green is the color associated with spring, but I do not believe that this has anything to do with Five Element Theory.

Some Qi Gong instructors say that when sending Qi to the Kidneys, one should think of blue or black and that when sending Qi to the Liver, one should hold the mental image of green in the mind. However, Five Element Theory in its original meaning simply referred to green as the color of Spring. Likewise other misinterpretations of color have crept in. Some people think that if you have a kidney problem, your facial complexion will be darker or that a liver problem will be manifested with a yellowish green facial color and that this problem will be worse in the Spring or on windy days.

In the face of the complexity of color interpretation, I believe that if one desires to concentrate on a color when transmitting Qi, it would be simplest to envision the basic color red while sending Qi anywhere in the body, whatever the condition of the patient who is being treated.

FIVE ELEMENT THEORY AND MEDICAL TREATMENT

1. I would recommend reading Chapter 10 (Acupuncture Channel Theory) prior to this section.

2. In modern Western medicine it is known that a disease of one organ can affect another, but not how to prevent this from happening or how to treat the problem after it has occurred.

From Five Element Theory we know that there are cycles of influence between the organs, as well as counteracting cycles where organs suppress or strengthen each other. Between these different cycles, one organ can affect all the others. However throughout history people have criticized Five Element theory as too mechanical and complicated. They have felt that it is often not clear how to put the theory into practice.

3. CONDITIONS

A) Chronic - One organ's chronic problem affects another organ. Using this concept we can deduce what has happened and predict what will occur next, but the prognosis of the patient is unclear.

B) Acute - People can have problems in two organs simultaneously. Emotional problems can exacerbate physical problems.

Using this information and Five Element Theory one can deduce the nature of the existing disease and which organ is affecting which other organs and then develop a treatment plan accordingly. But it will be difficult to determine the prognosis because there are so many possible interactions between different organs. For example, a problem with the Heart (Fire) can have either a tonifying or dispersing effect upon the Spleen (Earth). Likewise, via the controlling and counteracting cycles, the Heart can positively or negatively affect the Lungs (Metal).

Even this awkward and complex model of interactions between the organs is an improvement over traditional Chinese medical theories where, as in modern Western medicine, each organ problem or disease is treated individually with no consideration for its effect on the rest of the body. And even in today's most advanced forms of medicine much is still unknown when it comes to treatment.

Formulas for acupuncture treatment of patients were developed over time based on the Five Element classifications. About four hundred years ago these formulas were systematized and codified by a Korean Buddhist priest known to the world as Sa Am Do Yin, whose name can be translated as "cave dwelling Taoist." According to their code of ethics, Taoist and Buddhist priests never used their real names to gain fame as authors, so the true identity of this "cave dwelling Taoist" remains unknown. Nonetheless, Sa Am Do Yin has given the world formulas that remain popular in Korea, Japan and the West today.

Sa Am Do Yin's formulas are based on the internal flow of Qi between the organs. This means that his theory is more Yin in nature. My own Three Dimensional Four Inter-Channel Theory emphasizes the external flow of Qi through the channels. This is more Yang. Neither theory excludes or contradicts the other since external channel problems can become internal organ problems and internal disharmonies can manifest in the channels. Both approaches have their own advantages and their own truth. It is good to check both ways and to consider both treatment strategies.

For example, Sa Am Do Yin proposes the following: "If the Liver Channel acts excessively, sedate Heart 8." This point is selected because it is the Fire Point on the Fire Channel. Fire is the child of Wood, and this follows the principle "If Deficient, tonify the Mother. If Excess, disperse the Child."

In this case, I would suggest substituting Pericardium 8 for Heart 8. A Liver Channel problem can become a Heart Channel problem as Liver Fire becomes Heart Fire. But if you apply my Channel theory, you can see that Liver Channel problems can also block the Qi flow in the Gall Bladder, Triple Warmer, and Pericardium Channels. Therefore, I would prefer to use Pericardium 8, the Fire Point on the Pericardium Channel, for this problem (Jue Yin sister channel).

In another example, Sa Am Do Yin says "If the Gall Bladder Channel acts excessively, sedate Small Intestine 5." As in the previous example, the Fire Point on the Fire Channel is selected to treat Wood Excess. In this case it is a Yang Channel imbalance instead of Yin. But I would prefer to use Triple Warmer 6, also the Fire Point, because the Gall Bladder and Triple Warmer are paired Shaoyang brother Channels.

Formulas based on Five Element Acupuncture Theory use points between the knee and the foot for vertigo and eye problems cause by blockage of Qi circulation in the Gall Bladder Channel. However, using my Three Dimension Four Inter-Channel Theory and its "local-distant" hypothesis, I prefer to treat the local area where the Qi is stagnated. For instance, I will needle Gall Bladder 1 and Triple Warmer 17, two points on the head, along with more distant points such as Gall Bladder 37 and Triple Warmer 6.

Five Element Theory gives no explanation for Liver Channel Excess or Deficiency. But according to my own theory a statement like "Liver acts excessively" means either Liver Yang rising or Liver Fire rising. Sometimes symptoms of these disharmonies manifest in the Gall Bladder Channel with blood shot eyes and eye pain (Gall Bladder 1), temporal headache (GB 3, 4, 5, 6, 7 or 14), stiff neck (GB 12 and 20), and shoulder pain (GB 21).

This can happen in the case of hepatitis B or C when patients have not yet formed antibodies and also with gallstones. In these instances should one really treat these patients as "Liver Excess" or "Gall Bladder Excess"? I think not.

Finally I believe that Sa Am Do Yin, as a Taoist and Buddhist priest, no doubt had abundant Qi energy to call on as he healed patients using his formulas. But an ordinary acupuncturist without such abundant Qi may not be able to heal patients in the manner that he did if they follow his prescriptions automatically.

ELEMENT	WOOD	FIRE	EARTH	METAL	WATER
YIN CHANNELS					
Lung	LU 11	LU 10	LU 9	LU 8	LU 5
Heart	HT 9	HT 8	HT 7	HT 4	HT 3
Pericardium	PC 9	PC 8	PC 7	PC 5	PC 3
Spleen	SP 1	SP 2	SP 3	SP 5	SP 9
Kidney	K 1	K 2	K 3	K 7	K 10
Liver	Liv 1	Liv 2	Liv3	Liv 4	Liv 8

ELEMENT	METAL	WATER	WOOD	FIRE	EARTH
YANG CHANNELS					
Large Intestine	LI 1	LI 2	LI 3	LI 5	LI 11
Small Intestine	SI 1	SI 2	SI 3	SI 5	SI 8
Triple Warmer	TW 1	TW 2	TW 3	TW 6	TW 10
Stomach	ST 45	ST 44	ST 43	ST 41	St 36
Urinary Bladder	UB 67	UB 66	UB 65	UB 60	UB 40
Gallbladder	GB 44	GB 43	GB 41	GB 38	GB 34

Table 7-2

	TO TONIFY TO ORGAN'S FUNCTION IS DEFICIENT				TO SEDATE IF ORGAN'S FUNCTION IS EXCESSIVE			
	TONIFY		SEDATE		SEDATE		TONIFY	
Lung	LU 9	SP 3	LU 10	HT 8	LU 5	K 10	LU 10	HT 8
Large Intestine	LI 11	ST 36	LI 5	SI 5	LI 2	UB 66	LI 5	SI 5
Heart	HT 9	LIV 1	HT 3	K 10	HT 7	SP 3	HT 3	K 10
Small Intestine	SI 3	GB 41	SI 2	UB 66	SI 8	ST 36	SI 2	UB 66
Pericardium	PC 9	LIV 1	PC 3	K 10	PC 7	SP 3	PC 3	K 10
Triple Warmer	TW 3	GB 41	TW 2	UB 66	TW 10	ST 36	TW 2	UB 66
Spleen	SP 2	HT 8	SP 1	LIV 1	SP 5	LU 8	SP1	LIV 1
Stomach	ST 41	SI 5	ST 43	GB 41	ST 45	LI 1	ST 43	GB 41
Kidney	K 7	LU 8	K 3	SP 3	K 1	LIV 1	K 3	SP 3
Urinary Bladder	UB 67	LI 1	UB 40	ST 36	UB 65	GB 41	UB 40	ST 36
Liver	LIV 8	K 10	LIV 4	LU 8	LIV 2	HT 8	LIV 4	LU 8
Gallbladder	GB 43	UB 66	GB 44	LI 1	GB 38	SI 5	GB 44	LI1

Table 7-3

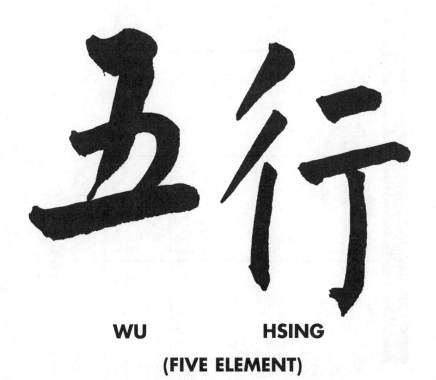

WU   HSING

(FIVE ELEMENT)

![Chapter 8]

Diagnostic Methods

A disease can be caused by only physical or psychological problems and most diseases are a combination of both. Many women suffer from temporal mandibular joint (TMJ) pain where they tend to clench their jaw or grind their teeth, usually during sleep. Some doctors will give their patients a rubber piece to bite down on while they sleep. Some dentists will recommend surgery to correct the joint. In doing this, they are only treating the symptom and not the cause. The same is true for people with digestive problems or ulcerative colitis. They can easily be treated with a proper diet and exercise. But while this reduces the symptoms, it does not address the problem, which in the United States is mostly due to stress. In the U.S., many people with psychological problems see a psychiatrist. Unfortunately, in many cases, the psychiatrist will prescribe drugs which only treat the symptom and not the cause. Oriental Medicine (holistic medicine) can be more effective than Western medicine because Oriental Medicine treats the patient as a whole. TMJ pain, stomach ulcers and ulcerative colitis are just a few examples of psychological rather than physical imbalance causing the problems which are treatable with acupuncture, herbs and meditation (Qi Gong breathing and Tai Chi).

What causes allergies? Eskimos living in the Arctic Circle region once traveled south to the Yukon River. When they entered areas where there were trees, grass and flowers, they started to sneeze and have runny noses and scratchy throats. This prompted them to move back up to the Arctic Circle. Soon after, their symptoms were gone. These days, Eskimos can travel further distances and can come in contact with modern facilities and goods because their allergies seem less severe. Once a family of Eskimos visited Los Angeles for a summer vacation and contacted a severe skin disease. Upon returning home, the disease dissipated. African Americans did not suffer from the same type of allergic symptoms as the Eskimos when they were brought to America. In Africa, there are many different kinds of plant life and dust patterns which helped their bodies to deal with different environmental conditions. These stories are not unlike the story told by Orsen Wells many years ago. The Martians, upon exposing themselves to a new environment, died from germs their bodies had never encountered and were not able to combat.

The examples above are commonly understood theories of allergies. People move to the United States from many different countries without any allergic reactions but there is no guarantee they will never suffer from allergies, even if they live in the same region with same pollution levels for several years. Switching from a day shift to a job on the night shift, a severe illness, mental stress such as divorce, death in the family, auto accident or bankruptcy might easily result in someone developing severe allergies. In many cases, the allergies will persist until the conditions which brought them on are removed. Typically, Western doctors would normally prescribe antihistamine for allergies. Practitioners of Oriental Medicine would do just the opposite and be certain the patient avoids any antihistamine product. Why? Because antihistamine depresses the Qi flow, which is the opposite of the treatment strategy of Oriental Medicine. Allergic reactions can be eliminated by dissolving the Qi and Blood stagnation and tonifying the Blood and Qi. This procedure is the main theory of Oriental Medicine. The practitioner of Oriental Medicine will instead treat the Qi and the Blood. This is an important aspect of Oriental Medicine: Diagnosis of any disease is always and simply a Qi or Blood stagnation or deficiency.

There are four important diagnostic methods which can be used depending on the experience and expertise of the doctor. These methods involve: 1) Visual observation, 2) Listening and olfactory skills, 3) Pulse taking and palpation of acupuncture points and 4) Asking the proper questions.

In most cases, you will probably not discover all the patient's problem during the first visit. It may take a few visits before you discover the nature of the problem the patient is suffering from.

Ayurvedic Medicine originated in India and has been practiced for thousands of years, predating Chinese medicine. Ayurvedic Medicine has similar techniques but primarily relies on tongue diagnosis and pulse taking.

1. VISUAL OBSERVATION

Much can be determined simply by looking at a person's body. Does the patient stand up straight or is he or she hunched over? Is the patient confident or shy? Skin color indicates the strength of the patient's Qi. Are there any skin or finger nail discoloration or disorders? Is there any discoloration or bruise around acupuncture points? Does the person have a long neck, which may lead to neck problems, or is the person heavy, which could bring on back troubles. The initial examination should be to observe the condition of the lips (for spleen), nose (for lung), eyes (for liver), ears (for kidney) and tongue (for heart).

The Oriental understanding of the spleen function is different than that of Western medicine. The spleen is covered more thoroughly in the Spleen section of Chapter 12.

The condition of the Lips will usually indicate the health of the Spleen

PALE: Cold and deficiency

RED: Heat

DRY: Dryness

BLUE/GREEN: Cold and stagnation

PURPLE: Congealing of blood, stagnation

CHAPPED: Spleen heat

TREMBLING OF LIPS, CANNOT CLOSE MOUTH: Spleen Qi deficiency

The condition of the Nose will usually indicate the health of the Lung

PURPLE: Cold

BLACK: Kidney Qi exhaustion

SWOLLEN: Spleen damp heat

WHITE: Lung Qi deficiency

DRY RED: Excess heat

The condition of the Eyes will usually indicate the health of the Liver.

UNCLEAR OR BLURRY: Dampness or Liver Qi deficiency and Blood deficiency

PURPLE: Liver wind (stroke)

TEARS, CRYING: Liver fire, anger, high blood pressure

SCALERA, WHITES OF EYES BECOME YELLOW : Jaundice, Liver Gall Bladder heat or Spleen damp heat

WIDE PUPILS: Drug over use

GRAY, DARKNESS, BAGS UNDER EYE: Kidney Qi deficiency

PROTRUDING: Phlegm and heat, thyroid problem

PHOTOPHOBIA: Excess Liver Qi

NEARSIGHTED/FARSIGHTED: Damp Liver, Kidney deficiency

Other body indicators include the ear which points towards the kidney conditions, the tongue for heart conditions and hair for energy and blood conditions.

When examining visually, you must be aware that there are many variables which may mislead you. For example, facial color may be hidden by makeup and lip color be changed with lipstick. Hair color or texture be changed with shampoo and dyes. Sometimes, you must check in places which are not usually altered, such as the palms.

Tongue Diagnosis

Observation of the tongue will provide clues to the health of the patient. Through the tongue, potential deficiencies in Yin, Yang, Qi or Blood can be identified. Signs to look for are color, texture, coating, size and any other abnormalities. A healthy tongue is normally pink or pale red. This may vary with each patient so it is important to ask what they may have noticed about their tongue in the past. Practitioners of Ayurvedic Medicine do tongue diagnosis much the same as other types of practitioners in Asia. A stroke patient usually suffers the effect of the stroke on one side of his or her body. The tongue will be thinner on the same side affected (see Figure 8-1).

It is easy to say that a pale tongue indicates Yang deficiency or a

CONDITION OF THE TONGUE	INDICATIONS
Pink or Pale Red	Normal
Pale	Yang Deficieny
Pale with Shiny Coat or no Coat	Blood & Yang Deficiency
Bright (Scarlet) Red	Yin Deficieny
Red & Moist	Damp & Heat or Yin Deficieny with Dampness or Lacking Internal Yang
Red & Dry	Yin Deficiency with Heat or Heart Fire Excess
Red on Both Sides	Liver & Gallbladder Heat
Red with Shiny Coat	Yin Deficiency in the Stomach
Red with Red Dots	Mild Heat in the Blood or Possibly Toxic Heat (Hepatitis)
Red with Purple Dots	Blood Stagnation or Blood Circulation Blocked by Heat
Red with White Dots	Heat with Qi Deficiency or Spleen & Stomach Deficiency
Purplish Red & Dry	Circulation Problems with Yin Damage
Dark Purple or Purplish & Moist	Blood Stagnation
Dark Purple or Purplish & Dry	Blood Stagnation & Extreme Heat
Dark Purple with Dry Coat	Damp Heat
Blue	Qi Stagnation or Liver Qi Stagnation or Yang Deficiency
Edema, Swollen Tongue with Teeth Marks	Yang Deficiency or Dampness or Yin Deficiency & Blood Deficieny
Cracks	Yin Deficiency or Congenital
Midline Crack*	Condition of Spine (Ayurvedic Medicine)

Table 8-1

TONGUE COAT	INDICATIONS
Yellow	Heat
White	Cold
Thick	Excess Stagnation
No Coat	Yin Deficieny
Coating Comes Off Easily	Weak Digestive System
Coating Does Not Come Off Easily	Healthy
Entire Coat Peels Off	Digestive System Yin
(Shiny Red Color)	is Depleated
Thick & Covers Entire Tongue	Excess Dampness of Phlegm
Thick, Sticky & Moist	Phlegm & Heat
Slippery, Moist & Wet	Dampness
Black Coating	Heat
Black Coating & Slippery or Wet	Coldness & Damp

Table 8-2

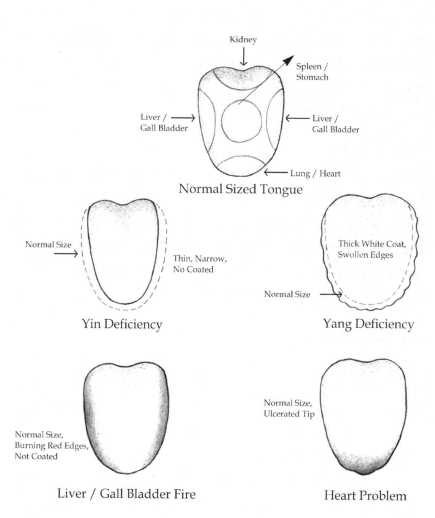

Kidney

Spleen /
Stomach

Liver /
Gall Bladder

Liver /
Gall Bladder

Lung / Heart

Normal Sized Tongue

Normal Size

Thin, Narrow,
No Coated

Yin Deficiency

Thick White Coat,
Swollen Edges

Normal Size

Yang Deficiency

Normal Size,
Burning Red Edges,
Not Coated

Liver / Gall Bladder Fire

Normal Size,
Ulcerated Tip

Heart Problem

Figure 8-1

red tongue may indicate Yin deficiency but it is not enough to just check the color. For example, if the tongue is red and dry, there may be a Yin deficiency with heat. The tables on page 8-1& 8-2 lists tongue conditions and what these conditions indicate. Remember, there are many parts of the body which will give hints as to what is wrong. The tongue is just one of many sign posts.

NAILS DIAGNOSIS

Much can be learned by observing the nail of a patent. A healthy nail is pink and has a shiny color. If the nail is excessively red, then there may be an over production of red blood cells. A pale nail indicates a blood deficiency. A yellowish color may be liver weakness and a bluish color means a lung and heart weakness (see Figure 8-2).

2. LISTENING/OLFACTORY

Emotional states can help determine certain internal problems. Listen to the patient's voice. A patient who speaks loudly or quickly may have high blood pressure, or anger. A person who speaks slowly or more softly may have low Qi levels. Just listening to how the patient describes symptoms will give clues to what the problem may be. Generally, a weak voice may indicate a deficiency in the lung Qi whereas a loud voice points towards liver excess. A healthy voice should be loud, sharp and clear.

Personal odors can also give signs as to the condition of the patient. Most people's sense of smell is not keen enough to detect body odors. However, as mentioned in Chapter 1, Taoist monks can develop a very acute sense of smell which helps them to diagnose patients. Personal odor will vary and change as the health of the individual changes.

PROBLEM ORGAN	LIVER	SPLEEN	LUNG	KIDNEY	HEART
SMELL	Rancid, smell of stale fat	Bad Breath	Fleshy smell	Putrid, decomposing, rotting, foul smell	Scorched smell

Table 8-3

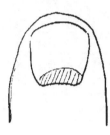

If Lower Portion of Nail

Bluish Color / Liver problom

Red Color / Heart Problem

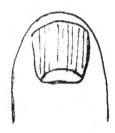

Vertical Lirues Indicake a Digestion problem

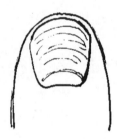

Horlzontal lines Indicate Malnutrition or chronic illness

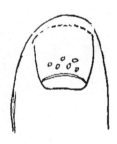

White Spots Inidicate a Calcium or Iron deficiencey

Fig. 8-2

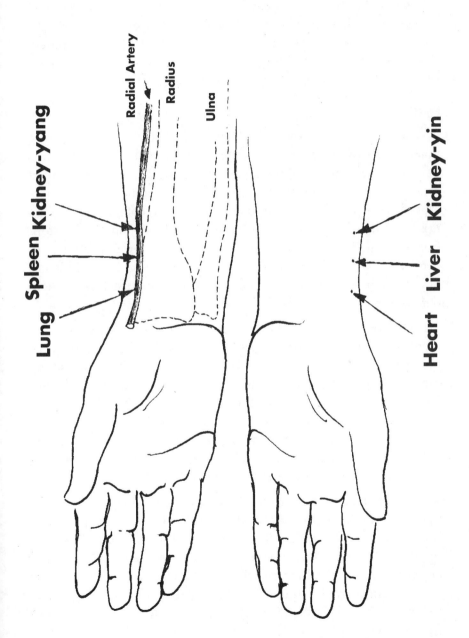

Fig. 8-3

3. PULSE TAKING AND PALPATION OF ACUPUNCTURE POINTS

PALPATION OF ACUPUNCTURE POINTS

Often, indications of where problems originate occur at acupuncture points. These points should be checked for bruised color, softness, nodules, or bumps. Each side must be checked and compared. These indicators will be discussed in Chapter 12, Treatment Methods. Acupuncture charts can be found in Chapter 10.

PULSE

When you walk into a doctor's office, you fill out a form asking you a series of questions about your medical past. A nurse leads you into an examination room where your body temperature, blood pressure and pulse are taken, usually with a machine. Then the doctor will come in a few minutes later and ask, "What's wrong?" Can this be enough? No. Let us look at the pulse for a moment. Western doctors will determine the health of the heart by the number of beats per minute. In Oriental Medicine, there are actually 18 levels of pulse to be checked and then over 50 different pulse types to help determine where the cause of illness may be.

Each wrist has three pulse points. The points on the right wrist identify the health of the lung, spleen and kidney Yang. The three points on the left wrist are indicators for the heart, liver and kidney Yin. Additionally, each pulse point has three different levels, Superficial, Middle and Deep. Studying the strength and feel or texture of each pulse point at different levels will help to determine whether the illness is related to external conditions or internal imbalance, and whether the imbalance is due to deficiency or excess in the Yin, Yang, Qi, Blood or a combination of these.

To check a pulse, sit across a table from the patient, placing the patient's hand and arm on the table, level with the heart, palm facing up. Place your middle finger on styloid process of radius as in Figure 8-3. Feel for the knob of a bone then move towards the lateral side of the radial artery where you can feel the pulse. Once your middle finger has found the pulse, place your index finger next to it nearer to the wrist and the ring finger on the other side, farther from the wrist.

The height of the patient determines the amount of space to be left between the fingers. A taller patient may require more space between the fingers. Roll your fingers onto the artery. Be certain to use the pad of your finger and not the tips so you do not confuse the patient's pulse with your own.

As mentioned earlier, there are three levels on which to check the pulse, Superficial, Middle and Deep. The superficial pulse is found at the surface of the skin with very little downward pressure from the fingers. The middle pulse can be found half way between the skin surface and the bone. The deep level pulse is found close to the bone.

A patient's condition can be determined by the type and depth of the pulse. A healthy pulse will feel smooth and occur with even frequency. It should feel powerful through the fingers. Finding a moderate pulse is very rare. Remember that pulse types vary by age, sex and body type. Even the weather and seasons can effect a pulse. For example, a superficial lung pulse is normal for autumn.

Diagnosing pulses is difficult at first. It may help to remember that pulse types can be divided into pairs — slow or rapid, deficient or excess, or in other words, Yin or Yang. The next section covers the most common types of pulses. Although the following descriptions may help in diagnosis, the practitioner must remember one thing — There is no substitute for experience. It will take many years before an acupuncturist can accurately diagnose a pulse.

MODERATE PULSE

A moderate pulse is a healthy pulse and is very rare. It is neither deep or superficial. All three fingers at the middle level feel even with normal strength and speed. Usually this kind of pulse is found in people after acupuncture treatment or Qi Gong practice. Typically, the right arm's pulse (lung, spleen and kidney Yang) will be weaker for men. With women and homosexual men, the left arm's pulse (heart, liver and kidney Yin) will be weaker.

Both men and woman over forty years of age will find that their kidney Yin and Yang pulses will get weaker over time.

PULSE DEPTH

SUPERFICIAL OR FLOATING PULSE

A superficial or floating pulse is an exterior and strong Yang pulse found just below the surface the skin. It moves along the surface of the skin, like a piece of wood floating on a stream. A superficial pulse often indicates that the body is fighting an exterior invasion such as a fever, chill or a headache. A deficient pulse can be felt on the surface but as you press down deeper, it fades and disappears like a ghost.

Wei Qi or defensive Qi travels outside organs, bones and arteries, protecting them from outside pernicious elements.

- If the Wei Qi is weak, then the superficial pulse will be weak. It is often accompanied by hot flashes and spontaneous sweating.

- If no floating pulse is found, the Wei Qi is too weak.

- If the Wei Qi is strong, the floating pulse will be strong.

- If the superficial pulse is weak but there are no external influences, then there is a Yin deficiency causing Yang to "float up."

Other floating pulse indications:

- If the pulse is floating and it feels slippery (longer) or slides by your fingers, it may indicate phlegm or mucous in the lung.

- A rapid floating pulse indicates heat in the lung.

- Lung and heart pulses which feel light and empty when you press down lightly and then disappear at the middle level may indicate deficient Qi and Blood or a loss of blood.

DEEP PULSE

A deep pulse moves through the bones and tendons and usually indicates the health of the kidney and liver. Like a stone sinking to the bottom of a river, you must go deep into the pulse to find clues. A deep pulse usually indicates a deficiency of the Yang. Qi and Blood are collecting at the interior and being obstructed or blocked from rising up. As mentioned before, the pulse's characteristics are influenced by the patient's body type. For a heavier or quiet person, a deep pulse is normal. Strength of spirit, mental, or emotional troubles can also be observed by checking the pulse.

Other deep pulse indicators:

- A deep and strong pulse shows that Qi is withdrawing from the outer surface of the body, often as a result of shock, pain or cold.

- A deep choppy pulse is a shorter pulse which feels as though it is having trouble getting through. If the pulse is weak and choppy, then stagnation of the Qi or Blood is most likely the problem.

- A deep, strong and choppy pulse indicates emotional suppression, trauma or excess blood stagnation.

PULSE SPEED

SLOW PULSE

As I indicated earlier, Western doctors measure the pulse by beats per minute. In fact, a more accurate method would be to measure pulse by breaths. A slow pulse is defined as one which has three beats per breath. It indicates a depletion of the Yang and is accompanied by symptoms of coldness as a result of slow blood circulation.

- If a pulse is slow and superficial, then the body is cold due to external forces.

- A deep slow pulse and chronic coldness are symptoms of Qi deficiency.

- A slow slippery pulse can indicate accumulation of cold phlegm or pregnancy.

- Choppy and slow pulses point to a blood deficiency.

- A slow and wiry pulse means that the pulse is being held inside, indicating Qi deficiency and liver Qi stagnation. This most often affects older people.

RAPID PULSE

A rapid pulse is one that has six beats per breath or 90 per minute. This is a symptom of excess heat in the system and an indication that the condition is acute. If the beat is more that 100 times per minute, then the patient is suffering from tachycardia.

If the pulse is rapid and thready, then there is a deficiency in the Yin (not to be confused with excess Yang).

A rapid and forceful pulse indicates true fire (extreme heat). Other symptoms associated with true fire are scanty urine, constipation or insomnia.

PULSE STRENGTH

DEFICIENCY PULSE

- A deficiency pulse is one that feels empty, like the stem of a scallion, and the Yang is weak. If the pulse is big, slow and soft and diminishes as you press deeper, then the sprit is depleted and Qi is low. Observe the patient's appearance and attitude for further confirmation.

- A pulse which disappears in the middle level indicates a Qi deficiency and an exhaustion of body fluid. In this case, the Qi does not have a foundation to rise up from, resulting in blood deficiency and a lack of nourishment. It may also be a result of summer heat.

Qi deficiency will appear as a weak superficial pulse which disappears when you press deeper. A blood deficiency will show a pulse which will be difficult to move around and will seem weak. A Yin deficiency causes a weak and rapid pulse where a Yang deficiency causes a slow and weak pulse.

EXCESS PULSE

An excess pulse is forceful and strong. It can be felt even at deep level by pressing hard. It is an acute symptom of any disease or may indicate Blood or Qi stagnation and sometimes an emotional problem such as excessive anger.

PULSE SIZE

BIG PULSE

This is a large diameter pulse indicating excess Yang or heat. If the pulse is big and weak and disappears as you press down, then there most likely a blood deficiency.

SMALL OR THREADY PULSE

This is a tiny diameter or slender pulse, thin like a string. It comes and goes with a definite shape. This indicates a deficiency in Yang or blood caused by an obstruction which forces everything to contract. If the pulse is small and rapid with heat, then there is a Yin deficiency.

PULSE LENGTH

LONG PULSE

A long pulse is healthy if the speed and strength are normal. Otherwise, it may indicate several different problems. Further examination of the pulse and the other indicators mentioned in the book must be undertaken to identify the problem.

SHORT PULSE

In general, a short pulse is a result of lung problems. A short weak pulse also indicates a Qi deficiency and a short strong pulse is a result of stagnation of the Qi in the middle jiao[33] (stomach, spleen).

PULSE TENSION

Relaxed Pulse

This is a healthy pulse, averaging four beats per breath. The pulse is easy going, comfortable, neither superficial nor deep. It is peaceful, signifying harmony in the spleen and stomach.

TIGHT PULSE

A patient with pain or coldness may have this type of pulse. This pulse is tense and sharp and feels strong with pressure. A tight pulse is the result of a contraction of the blood vessels. It feels similar to a wiry pulse and is an internal imbalance of Yin and Yang, as result of the blood not being nourished.

PULSE SMOOTHNESS

CHOPPY PULSE

This pulse feels like scraping bamboo twigs with a knife and does not flow smoothly. This type of pulse indicates either blood stagnation or Jing or blood deficiency.

SLIPPERY PULSE

This type of pulse is smooth and forceful. It can be due to excessive dampness and phlegm retention in the body. Sometimes, people with abundant Qi and blood will show this type of pulse. A slippery pulse can usually be found in pregnant women as well. This is pulse feels the opposite of a choppy pulse.

WIRY PULSE

When you press down with your fingers, the pulse feels like the blood is not moving and is as tight as an extended bowstring. A wiry pulse usually indicates liver Qi stagnation. Typically, the patient will feel angry and will be very emotional.

MISSED BEAT

A missed beat is exactly that; the pulse feels as though it is skipping a beat. The regularity or irregularity of the skipped beat is an important clue to the cause of the problem. This type of pulse usually indicates heart problems and may be congenital.

SYMPTOMS AND THE PULSE TYPE THAT WILL RESULT FROM COLD

Cold Obstruction: Deep, forceful

Internal Cold Obstruction: Deep, slow, deficient

Deep and Hidden Cold: Strong or weak

SYMPTOMS AND THE PULSE TYPE THAT WILL RESULT FROM HEAT

True Fire: Superficial, strong, rapid

Summer Season: Floating pulse at all levels

Yin deficiency, Heat: Rapid, superficial, weak

Liver Yang or fire rising: Choppy, rapid, strong or wiry

SYMPTOMS AND THE PULSE TYPE THAT WILL RESULT FROM PAIN

Deep, Excess, Wiry, rapid, tight, contraction

FIXED STABBING PAIN

Short, strong

INDICATIONS OF YANG DEFICIENCY

Deep, Slow

DEFICIENCY

Thready, Short

INDICATIONS OF YIN DEFICIENCY

Rapid, Thready, Deficient, Short

4. QUESTIONING

What is Wrong?

In the United States, people are used to going to doctors and telling them what is wrong. This is helpful but in most cases, Doctors of Western Medicine focus only on the specific problem the patient mentions. Doctors of Western medicine can only treat what they can see. If drugs will not cure the problem, they will often resort to surgery. What these doctors do not understand is that most illnesses originate in one place but manifest themselves in another, giving the doctor a false indication of where the problem really lies. In Asia, patients often do not even tell their doctor what the problem is. They simply stop in and say "what's wrong with me?" Often, there won't even be a problem. The patient just comes in for a check up.

When meeting a patient, the first question to ask is obviously about his or her main complaint. The thoroughness of your questions will ultimately decide whether you properly diagnose the patient. The patient will usually not tell you all the information you need to know, just what he or she thinks you need or want to know. If a patient's main complaint is chills, he or she might not think to tell you about other symptoms, such as pain on the bottom of the foot, because the patient does not think that this is related to the main symptom. Pain on the bottom of the foot is a sign of a Kidney problem or Kidney Yang deficiency which may result in chills. Listen carefully not only to what the patient says, but how he or she says it, listen to the voice and watch the body language. There are sixteen categories of questions you must investigate. They are listed below with some examples of the questions you might ask. Also, refer to Chapter 4 for additional information on what causes disease.

MAIN COMPLAINT:

• Why has the patient come to the clinic?

TEMPERATURE

• Does a patient prefer hot or cold water or food?

• Which season does the patient prefer?

• Does the patient feel hot or cold — feet, hands, head, stomach, etc.?

PERSPIRATION

Does he or she perspire? If so, when and where? If a little exertion causes perspiration, then a Qi deficiency may be present. Perspiration at night indicates Yin deficiency. If this is the case, then the patient's hands and feet may begin to perspire about 1/2 hour after falling asleep. It is important to remember that weakness due to surgery may cause perspiration after only a few steps of walking. Interview the patient thoroughly.

PAIN

• Where is the pain?

• Does the patient feel dizzy or have spasms? When and where?

• Describe the pain. Is it sharp, dull, shooting etc.?

• What relieves the pain and what makes it worse — hot cold, pressure, etc.?

Remember that pain is often a symptom. Pain in the right side may indicate that there is a tumor or an abnormality on the left side of the spine. When investigating pain, the doctor must keep in mind that if a condition has been chronic for a long period of time, numbness may occur, blocking any pain that might normally be felt.

DIGESTION

• Ask about the patient's appetite.

• What type of foods does the patient like — hot, cold, spicy etc.?

• What flavors and tastes appeal to the patient?

• What is hard to digest?

• If the patient has digestion problems, when does he or she feel the worst (time of day or which meal)?

SLEEP

- How much sleep does the patient get?

- What time does he or she wake up during the night?

- Does the patient feel rested after sleep?

- Does the patient have trouble falling asleep? This may indicate Yin deficiency or emotional problems.

REPRODUCTIVE ORGANS

- Is menstruation regular or painful?

- Is the menstruation cycle shorter than 28 days (Yin deficiency or false heat) or longer than 28 days (Yang deficiency with cold or Qi deficiency)?

- During menstruation, if the blood color is dark or brown, then blood stagnation is indicated.

- PMS (Pre Menstrual Syndrome) — Is it emotional, physical, or both?

- Has the level of sexual energy changed?

- Is there Leukorrhea?

- Is the patient impotent?

- Is there pain anywhere in the area (uterus, ovaries or testicles)?

PHYSICAL INJURIES

Does the patient have any:

- Spinal damage?

- Sports injuries?

- Surgical scars?

- Problems with joints (neck, back, knees, etc.)?

Ailments caused by physical injuries are primarily an American phenomenon. Americans are more athletic than Asians, so their injuries tend to be more physical or external in nature.

• Are there any other discharges (mucus, blood, etc.)?

• Where is the pain?

• Does the patient have constipation or diarrhea?

URINE

Check the color of the urine. If it is dark yellowish, the patient has heat. Clear urine indicates cold. Frequent, urgent, and painful urination may indicate a kidney and/or a bladder infection. If the patient needs to urinate frequently at night during the winter, there may be a Yang deficiency.

Ayurvedic Medicine collects urine samples for color, bubbles, or smell, whereas the Chinese does not.

BREATHING

• Does the patient cough a lot? At what time of day?

• Does the patient have asthma?

• Listen to the patient's breathing — Is it heavy, light, regular, etc.?

• Is there shortness of breath? This sometimes may indicate heart problems.

VISION/HEARING

• Is there twitching of the eye?

• Are the eyes blood shot, indicating liver Yang or fire?

• Is there double vision, indicating a gall bladder channel problem?

• Does the patient have difficulty hearing which may be due to kidney Yang deficiency?

• Does the patient suffer from tinnitus (ringing in the ear)?

If the patient hears a high pitched sound, there may be Yin deficiency with false heat or liver fire rising. This type of problem can occur after menopause. If the patient hears a low pitched ringing, this may be caused by a kidney/spleen Yang Qi deficiency.

EMOTIONAL PROBLEMS

As mentioned earlier, the source of a patient's problem may be physical or psychological. Check for:

- Childhood emotional scars
- Death in the family
- Divorce
- Bankruptcy
- Job loss

FAMILY MEDICAL HISTORY

It is also important to determine if the patient may have inherited the illness. Check for:

- Diseases or illnesses in the past
- Hereditary diseases or illnesses

LIVING CONDITIONS

A patient's living conditions will always affect their health. This may not be as much of a problem in the United States as it is in China since the living conditions in the U.S. are usually high and uniform where ever a patient may go. In America, you need to ask where the person has come from, whether a different part of the United States or another county. Also ask how long the patient lived in each region, since environmental conditions will vary in the North, South, East or West. Find out about the environment the patient lived:

- Dry or damp?
- Windy?
- Cold or warm?

Exposure to harmful environmental factors such as lead paint is also important.

OCCUPATIONAL CONDITIONS

A person working in a factory may be exposed to a lot of dust, chemicals, or fibers. Perhaps the area the person works in is not suited for his or her body. For example, if a cook works at a table which is too high or too low, he or she could develop carpal tunnel syndrome. Many modern office buildings have very poor air circulation. Often, the air conditioning system may cause the office to be too warm or too cold.

LIFE STYLE

Usage of alcohol, tobacco, and drugs will all have an effect on a patient's health. Find out if the patient exercises and if so, what type of exercise is done.

YIN/YANG THEORY

The Yin and Yang theory in Chapter 6 covers the theory in general. In this section, I would like to describe how the Yin/Yang theory operates in the human body.

Yin represents femininity, liquid, blood, body moisture, passivity, calmness and peace of mind. Yang, on the other hand, represents masculinity, body warmth, vitality, high activity, libido and aggressiveness.

While comparisons are not absolute, it is useful to make them to better understand Yin/Yang theory. Children, for example, are more Yang than adults since they have more body warmth and are more active. As men get older, they lose their Yang energy, usually from stress or sexual activity. As women get older, they lose their Yin energy, usually from menstruation, child birth and in particular, immediately after giving birth. People over 60 years-old lose both Yin and Yang energy.

The following syndromes, Yang excess, Yin deficiency, Yin excess and Yang deficiency are discussed below. Not all the symptoms mentioned are necessary to determine a patient's illness. Some patients may exhibit all the symptoms while others display only a few. The symptoms may also vary in degrees of severity from patient to patient.

YANG EXCESS

Yang excess is often referred to as True Heat. People with this type of affliction will have a severe aversion to heat. Typically, this excess Yang or heat is only temporary and will go away after a few days. However, if it does persist for too long, severe damage may result due to the Yin deficiency and may in some cases, cause death. Death will occur when the Yin has been totally depleted.

Symptoms of Yang excess are dark scanty urine, sweating, fatigue, constipation and insomnia. The tongue will be red with a thick yellow coat. The pulse will be rapid, large and strong. If the Yang excess is acute, severe and lasts more than a few days, then the patient will experience excessive sweating and the body will be red with heat. Some patients experience delirium and will feel a great deal of pain when touched or massaged (see Figure 8-4).

YIN DEFICIENCY

Yin deficiency (false heat) is usually chronic and shows symptoms of heat. However, it is the lack of Yin which causes this type of heat instead of Yang excess. Yin deficiency is also referred to as Tidal Fever since the patient will experience hot flashes or periods of hot and cold like the tide coming in and out. As you might expect, Yin deficiency has some of the same symptoms as Yang excess. The patient will dislike heat, have dark urine, feel tired, have insomnia, and experience constipation. There are some different symptoms as well. The tongue will be red, thin, and narrow with no coat. The pulse will be rapid but weak. Women will find that their menstrual cycle will shorten, often occurring every 26, 25, or 24 days instead of 28. In cases where the problem is chronic, the patient will have night time sweating. There will be hot flashes on the cheeks, the bottoms of the feet, the palms and sometimes the chest. The throat will be dry. As with Yang excess, people with Yin deficiency will have a strong aversion to being touched. Pre-existing joint stiffness, pain, or neuralgia may be worsened by a Yin deficiency. The patient can drink a fair amount of water to help the joint pain caused by dehydration, but this will do nothing to resolve the Yin deficiency (see Figure 8-5).

YIN EXCESS

Yin excess is extremely rare. If coldness attacks the patient, he or she will have cold limbs and a pale face. The urine will be clear and scanty. The pulse will be slow and strong and the tongue will be pale with a thick white coat. In acute cases, the patient will have temporary spells of diarrhea and a feeling of heaviness, and will not want to be touched in the stomach area. There may also be a feeling of dampness. This can be caused by consuming a lot of cold food or drink in hot weather. Yin excess will consume Yang Qi and if it is severe and continues over a long period of time, it will cause Yang deficiency (see Figure 8-6).

YANG DEFICIENCY

This is also usually a chronic condition where the patient will experience symptoms of coldness. Patients with Yang deficiency will have a very low energy level. Their limbs will be cold and their faces will be pale. They will have clear but profuse urine. (This may be attributed to a kidney Yang deficiency.) They may also have edema. Their pulse will be slow and weak and their tongue will be pale, flabby, and have a white coat. There may also be teeth marks on the tongue. In chronic cases, the patient may experience diarrhea in the morning, often around 6:00 a.m. The slightest exertion will cause the patient to sweat. Whereas with Yang excess, the patient will be very tired and suffer from insomnia, a patient with Yang deficiency will be very sleepy, sleeping 10 hours or more a day. The patient will catch colds easily and does not mind being massaged. Often, patients with Yang deficiency will feel very good after Qi Gong massage. Libido and sexual desire and energy will be weakened (see Figure 8-7).

CAUSES OF YIN AND YANG EXCESSES AND DEFICIENCIES

There are many theories as to why excesses and deficiencies in Yin and Yang occur. My research has shown that there are several external and internal factors which effect Yin and Yang. Weather, emotion and foods are a few examples.

Take for example the 55 year-old widow who is going through

menopause. She took a summer vacation from Boston to Miami Beach in Florida. The air conditioners in her beach house and her car were broken. It was so muggy and hot that she became irritable and angry. The hot weather and anger consumed more Yin. There were no other cars to rent and the rental agency could not repair her car until the next day. The agent who rented the beach house to her had no others available and the air conditioner repair man did not work on Sunday. So, she purchased an airline ticket to Alaska. During the flight, the air plane encountered engine trouble and made an emergency landing on a glacier. She was wearing only her summer clothes and was frightened and cold. This consumed a lot of her Yang energy and left her shivering and hungry. A Korean gentleman sitting next to her opened a gift box and took out a large piece of Korean ginseng root and offered it to her with a glass of whiskey. His kindness and warmth cheered her up (increasing her Yang energy). The whiskey and ginseng root raised her levels of Yang Qi.

The story above is just an example of how the environment and the foods we eat can effect Yin and Yang levels. Joy and happiness will increase Yang levels while sadness and depression will lower Yang levels. Often when a person feels happiness and joy, they will have a lot of energy. They will want to go out and celebrate, feeling the need to move and keep going. On the other hand, a person who is sad or depressed will have low energy, wanting to just sit or sleep.

Hot temperatures will increase Yang and consume Yin while cool temperatures will decrease Yang or consume Yang energy. During the summer, people will generally have more energy, wanting to go out and do things where during the winter months, people will be less energetic.

Hot or spicy foods will increase Yang and cooler foods will decrease Yang. Changes in Yin or Yang due to food are more noticeable internally. Hot spicy food will cause the person to sweat whereas cool foods may cause chills.

Emotion, food, and weather will not cause excess conditions. They will just change the balance of Yin and Yang. Incorrect medical treatment will also affect Yin and Yang levels. For instance, it is assumed that taking ginseng root is an effective way to increase

Yang levels. This is only half true. Korean ginseng will increase Yang and energy levels but American ginseng does the opposite, increasing Yin energy.

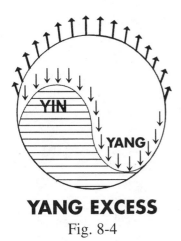

YANG EXCESS

Fig. 8-4

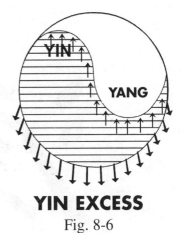

YIN EXCESS

Fig. 8-6

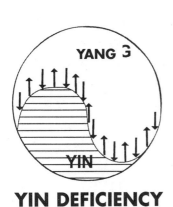

YIN DEFICIENCY

Fig. 8-5

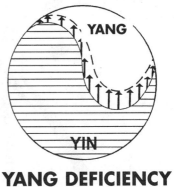

YANG DEFICIENCY

Fig. 8-7

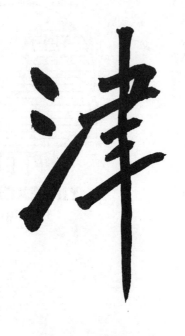

JIN

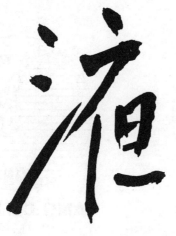

YE

BODY FLUID

Chapter 9

Various Treatment Methods of Oriental Medicine

The treatment principle of Oriental Medicine is to balance Yin and Yang, resolve Qi stagnation and relieve Qi deficient patients by the following methods:

- Acupuncture Treatment
- Moxa Treatment
- Cupping
- Qi Gong Massage
- Qi Gong exercise (martial arts)
- Meditation
- Diet Therapy
- Folk Medicine
- Herbal Medicine

Each civilization has developed its own treatments based upon the herbs available to them. Treatment techniques will vary according to many factors such as diet and climate.

ACUPUNCTURE TREATMENT

Within each of us, there exists a complex network of sensitivity points that link the surface of our bodies to our internal organs and to certain physical behavioral patterns. Through these internal "channels" of energy flow our life force or Qi. Disease can often be attributed to a blockage of Qi, and the acupuncturist treats disorders by inserting super-thin needles into the appropriate points to release Qi flow.

Acupuncture is most effective when treating acute problems such as severe pain or a heat condition such as fever. Acupuncture works faster than moxa (which is discussed in the next section) and acupuncture treatment strengthens or energizes Qi and blood flow which in turn increases the body's ability to fight disease.

There have been nine different types of acupuncture needles used throughout history. The type of needle used will depend upon where the needle is to be inserted. Needles will vary in size and composition. In Japan, Korea and America, acupuncturists often use thin needles with insertion tubes. Some Chinese still use very long needles. Modern acupuncture needles are disposable and are so thin as to not be painful when inserted.

After acupuncture treatment, the health of the blood and lymphatic systems will improve. The immunities of the body are increased and the secretion of internal hormones is better controlled.

MOXA/MOXIBUSTION

Moxibustion is a method for treating and preventing diseases through the application of heat to certain acupuncture points. Moxa is usually found in the shape of a cigar and is made of mugwort leaves (Folium Artemisia Argyi).

As mentioned earlier, acupuncture is very effective when curing acute problems. Moxa generates a great deal of heat, and when applied near or on the skin surface, helps to relieve channel obstructions caused by dampness or cold. Moxibustion is effective in curing chronic problems such as stomach problems or indigestion, coldness, numbness and weakness. Moxa is a tonification method which can be used by everyone.

After moxibustion, the white and red corpuscles and the body's immunity to disease are increased. The revival ability of cellular tissue is improved as after an injection of protein. Blood circulation, absorption of nutrition, bodily function and metabolism are improved as is the skeletal strength.

The ways to apply moxa include through a moxa cone, moxa stick or on the head of an acupuncture needle. It can be applied either directly or indirectly. In the case of a moxa cone, lit moxa is placed directly on the skin. Depending on the nature of the disease, the moxa can be left on the skin to cause a burn or can be removed and replaced with another cone if the first one gets too hot (Figure 9-1). To apply a moxa cone indirectly, the doctor will cover the point with a slice of ginger, garlic or salt. A moxa stick is applied by bringing the lit moxa close to the skin then moving it away (Figure 9-2). Placing a lit piece of moxa on an acupuncture needle is the third method of application (Figure 9-3).

How to Apply Moxa Stick

When purchasing moxa, I recommend the smokeless type which is made of mugwort leaves (Folium Artemisiae Argyi). This is usually 1/4 inch diameter and 4 1/2 inches long. First, wrap the stick with aluminum foil to prevent an unwanted smell on your fingers. Second, light the moxa stick with a cigarette lighter, or the flame on a stove. It will take a few minutes before the moxa will start to burn. Third, warm the acupuncture point or asi[34] points. To keep from accidentally burning yourself, use your edge of the palm as a guide by placing it near the spot you are treating (see Figure 9-2). Place the burning moxa about an inch from the skin above the acupuncture point. Do not hold it stationary, move the moxa around a circle of 1 inch diameter. Do this for a few seconds until the skin starts to feel hot then move to another point. Make sure you tap the stick to shake-off loose ashes to prevent accidental burning. Treat yourself with moxa for about 15 minutes on both the front and back of your body. If your condition is acute or chronic and time allows, apply moxa two or three times a day. In an emergency such as severe indigestion or a heart attack, use warm water on the hands and feet first and then apply moxa to the hands and feet. Then treat the front points around the abdomen. After treatment, extinguish the moxa fire with water and let dry for a few days. Use another moxa stick alternately.

You do not need to know exactly where the acupuncture point is. Moxa anywhere near the points will be effective in moving Qi and blood stagnation in your body (see Figure 9-1, Figure 9-2 and Figure 9-3).

Cupping

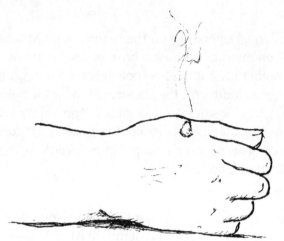

Fig. 9-1

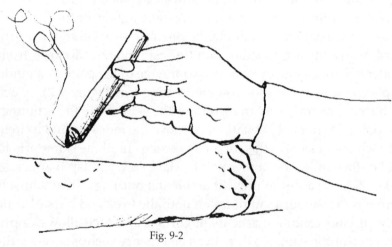

Fig. 9-2

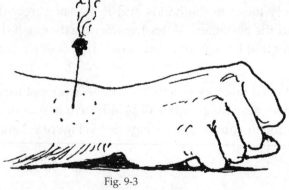

Fig. 9-3

The cupping method is most often used in the Middle East and Europe. This method involves igniting a cotton ball soaked in alcohol. The lit cotton is placed inside a glass, bamboo or plastic cup, heating the air inside. The cup is then placed on the skin and held in place by the suction caused by the vacuum, which creates heat suction on the surface of the skin. The Japanese have developed a modern method of cupping. It involves placing a glass cup over an area of the skin. Through the use of a small hand pump attached to a valve on the top of the cup, a suction is created on the skin surface.

QI GONG MASSAGE

In the west, massage concentrates primarily on the muscles. However massage should be applied to the entire body. The most effective method for applying Qi Gong massage is to put Qi into the patient. A Qi Gong massage therapist will concentrate on the body's channels, moving the patient's Qi and applying Qi at key points of the body. Qi Gong massage should not be confused with Shiatsu, a massage therapy developed in Japan. Shiatsu can be an effective method for moving Qi, but the practitioner's Qi can leak out through his or her fingers and the kneeling position of the practitioner can cause Qi stagnation and imbalance in the patient as well.

QI GONG EXERCISE (MARTIAL ARTS)

Qi Gong is a Chinese system of breathing and exercises used for personal health, healing and therapy. It is an internal method of practice and a skill used by martial artists for protection and power. Using Qi Gong, healers can create intense energy and externalize and transfer their Qi flow. Qi Gong combined with traditional acupuncture is perhaps the most potent of all treatments.

MEDITATION

There are many different types of meditation. These types of techniques will be the subject a later book.

DIET THERAPY

Western nutritional experts are concerned with the amount of vitamins, fiber, etc., that people consume daily. Oriental therapy has a different approach to a balanced diet. There are a large number of Oriental remedial cooking therapies designed to treat health problems.

One of the most popular therapies is the time honored tradition of chicken soup with medicinal herbs. Ordinary or Chinese black bone chicken soup with ginseng root or Huang Qi (astragali root) is well known in the Orient. Even modern nutritionists agree that boiled chicken without the skin is one of the best low-fat protein sources available.

An Oriental herbal doctor may prescribe a formula consisting of animal parts or organs made into a soup with herbs. For thousands of years in the Orient, people ate corresponding animal organs if their own organs were diseased. Now we can extract the vitamins and hormones from organs of an animal. Most Taoists, however, will not use animal parts in their treatment for ethical considerations.

Another traditional recipe is seaweed soup. For thousands of years Korean women have eaten seaweed soup for a month after giving birth. Tradition has it that they learned to do this while observing a female whale eat a great amount of seaweed after delivering a baby whale. Modern research substantiates this behavior. Seaweed contains a large amount of iodine, an element always lacking in the system of post partum women.

As with all therapies, indiscriminate eating can aggravate a situation. If a woman takes ginseng tea, cinnamon, ginger, pepper, onions or lamb chops when she has high blood pressure, fever, or hot flashes due to menopause it will only make the situation worse. These substances increase blood pressure, promote vaginal bleeding between menses, cause more hot flashes, constipation and insomnia.

A person who is feeling cold in the body because of Yang deficiency and has low energy, poor appetite, indigestion, and nausea, will have his or her condition aggravated by eating fresh fruits and seafood or being on a long-term vegetarian diet.

FOLK MEDICINE

Folk medicine is not well organized and systematized as are

Chinese or Ayurvedic Medicine. But it has been used for centuries by country folks to cure local ailments. Sometimes it works and sometimes not. It is likely that folk medicine was the basis for herbal medicine. The difference between folk medicine and herbal medicine is that folk medicine only involves one herb whereas an herbalist may prescribe a mixture of herbs. Also, herbalists are trained to differentiate diseases to determine the best remedy.

- Radish seed - In Korea, the radish seed is said to cure indigestion.

- Crushed Freshwater Snail Shells - Helps acidic stomach pain.

- Clay - In Africa as well as in Korea, it is widely believed that the cure for an infection is to put clay on the affected area. There is also a reference to folk medicine in the life of Jesus Christ who is said to have spit on the ground, mixed it with dirt and placed the dirt mixture on the eye of a blind man to cure his blindness. This is known as antibiotic medicine. Several kinds of Mycin come from streptomyces bacteria, which is found in soil.

- Dried Ginger - This was used to cure nose bleeds. The doctor would burn the skin of dried ginger then put it into the patient's nostrils.

- Pomegranate - Cut out the root of a pomegranate that grows towards the east. Fry and dry it, then boil and drink the tea. This was the cure for Amenorrhea (lack of menstruation) or tapeworm.

- Pepper - If you were bitten by a centipede, you were told to chew a pepper leaf and mix it well with saliva, then place it on the skin where you got bit.

- Cherry - Make cherry leaf juice and drink a small cup of tea five times a day. Pound the cherry root that grows in an easterly direction and put it on the skin to cure a snake bite.

- Peach Leaves and Nicotine - Put the resin collected from a cigarette pipe in the nose of a snake and you can get it to faint. Put the peach leaves in the nose to revive it.

In some of the examples mentioned above, only roots of plants growing in an easterly direction are used. This is actually a Taoist tradition, formulated by observing insects and snakes.

HERBAL MEDICINE

Most ancient cultures knew that nature, through the earth, provided all the medicine we needed. Chinese, Persian, Korean, Indian, African, American Indian and Middle Eastern civilizations have used herbal medicine throughout their history to treat specific disorders or to tonify their bodies for perfect health. Over the centuries, the observation and deduction of Asian herbalists have refined these methods to a system that uses over 1,000 herbs, plants and animal parts.

Thousands of years ago in Korea, certain tribes worshipped bears. Taoists observed sick bears and recorded which herbs or minerals they ate for a remedy. For many years, these herbs were imported to Korea from China, making them very expensive and available only to the wealthy nobles. About 400 years ago, a Korean doctor named Huh Jun began research on herbs native to Korea. As explained in Chapter One, a Taoist has the ability to communicate with or understand animal calls and sounds. They can detect the type of sickness or disease and where it is in the animal's body. Huh Jun would observe the diet of sick bears in hope of learning about natural medicines using local herbs. Unfortunately, he did not follow the Taoist ways and would often become very sick from the herbs he tested.

Where folk medicine used a single substance for a simple symptom, Chinese herbal therapy used from four to thirty different kinds of herbs combined to treat anything from a simple symptom to complex syndromes. In modern times, the Chinese tend to use large dosages of herbs if it seems to fit the patient's aliment. The Korean style of herbal medicine is to use a small dosage each time. This treatment method, used by herbalists who treated the nobility, emphasized caution. These herbalists were the founders of the Modern College of Korean Traditional Medicine. The Japanese take very small amounts of herbs, similar to the small portions they eat in their meals. Early in the 1960's, the Japanese developed a method of taking herbal extracts and mixing them to make herbal formulas. The idea of taking pills, however, never caught on because Asians prefer direct decoction of herbal medicine.

Modern researchers in Asia, Europe and America have been analyzing herbs chemically and have been testing these on animals and people. Modern experience in using these herbs is limited when compared to Oriental herbs which have been taken by hundreds of millions of people over thousands of years. The United States Food and Drug Administration (FDA) classifies herbs as health foods and not medicine. This policy should be changed because classifying herbs as medicine would lead to greater enforcement and ultimately, a safer product. If you take a modern medicine that uses herbs, be sure to consult your herbalist first. Your herbalist should be fairly fluent in English and should have at least a four-year college degree in Oriental Medicine. He or she should also be licensed by the state you reside in.

Sometimes people ask about new herbal products with fancy claims from Africa, South America and elsewhere. Some readers may remember Comfrey, a popular herb in the 1970's until the FDA warned that too much of it would cause liver cancer. Comfrey has been banned completely in Germany. Once many health food companies claimed fish oil could lower cholesterol levels and high blood pressure, but FDA research found that there was no scientific basis for these claims. Any new drug or herb can have a good or bad effect. In the early 60's Cortisone was the miracle drug of choice for joint pain. Now it is considered hazardous to receive more than three injections of Cortisone into a joint or muscle as it will damage and harden the area permanently. We still hear about the different effectiveness of aspirin today.

There are many different herbal formulas. My upcoming book on herbal medicine will cover herbal formulas to treat some of the more common ailments found today. These formulas are modified to fit American lifestyles, stress levels, and eating habits. I have been developing these herbal formulas in a capsule form using a lower dosage of ingredients. Insects, snakes, or other animal parts (except deer antler) are not used as I follow Taoist traditions by not using animal parts as it seems unethical.

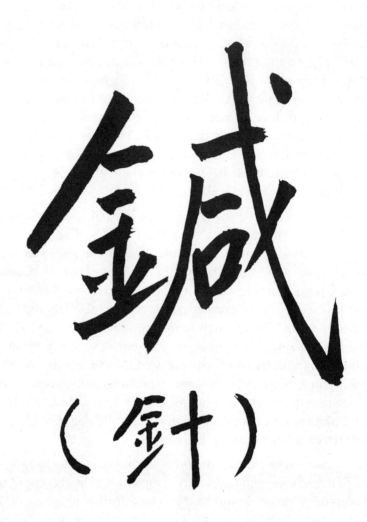

CHEN(ACUPUNCTURE)

Chapter 10

Acupuncture Channel Theory

Most acupuncturists will say that Oriental Medicine is holistic and that any one problem in the body can affect the entire body both physically and emotionally. This is undoubtedly true. As I mentioned in Chapter 6 on Yin/Yang Theory, the Western Cartesian system and Eastern Yin/Yang theory look at the world in a radically different manner. Yin/Yang theory, unlike the rigid limits of the Cartesian coordinate system, has boundaries that are fluid and permeable and sees the universe as an unbroken wholeness, as David Bohm has written. [35] Qi flow can be influenced not only by what is happening in and around the body, but even by the sun, the moon, and forces from other planets. But how many acupuncturists are really able to apply this perspective in the treatment of their patients as they claim to do?

Too many acupuncturists treat only symptoms, just as Western medicine does. For example, when treating a patient with carpal tunnel syndrome, one needs to check not only the wrist area, but also the elbow and neck, and on the lower limb both the ankle and knee on the same side. In order to understand why and how to do this, my interchannel theory must be applied both for diagnosis and to design the treatment method.

Determining prognosis is the most difficult task in medicine, whether the practitioner is trained in the Oriental or Western approach. As I mentioned in Chapter 7 on Five Element Theory, trying to apply this style to determine prognosis becomes too complicated because there are simply too many possibilities. Any physical organ problem can affect all the other organs. (This is not the case with long-term emotional problems which disturb only a certain organ.) To understand how to use this system properly to treat patients is not simple and straightforward.

Myung Kim's Three Dimensional Four Inter-Channel Theory

I believe that my own acupuncture interchannel theory can be used to determine the prognosis of the patient more effectively than any other system that I am aware of. I have developed my system over my many years of practicing martial arts, researching, and treating patients in my clinic. I think that I have rediscovered the meaning and significance of the interchannel relationships defined as Tai Yang, Shao Yang, Yang Ming, Tai Yin, Shao Yin, and Jue Yin. To properly understand these interrelationships can be very useful in diagnosis, prognosis, and treatment. This chapter is designed to help you do this effectively (refer to Figures 10-1, 10-2, 10-3).

Figure 10-4 shows the flow of Qi through the channels of the human body over a 24-hour period. Qi flow follows a regular course throughout the body with maximum flows through given acupuncture channels and their corresponding organs occurring during a two-hour interval. Since blood flow follows Qi, there will also be an increase in the blood carried to the affected organ during this period. This increased Qi and blood flow can explain symptoms reported by patients occurring during these periods of peak flow.

Since peak Qi flow through the Heart Channel and the heart itself occurs between 11 a.m. and 1 p.m., there can be an increased likelihood of heart attacks at noon time. The heart may be weakened by disease or congestion and may not be able to handle the increased blood flow following the Qi. Heart attacks can, of course, occur at any time of the day, and there are many cases of heart patients suffering attacks upon wakening to the sound of an alarm clock. This is because the heart is particularly sensitive to sudden sounds, and attacks at this hour have nothing to do with increased Qi flow.

Peak Qi flow to the Lung Channel and the lungs occurs between 3 and 5 a.m., and there is increased likelihood of severe coughing occurring in otherwise mild cases of asthma around 4 a.m. Of course, patients with chronic or severe asthma conditions may experience asthma attacks at any time of the day.

Peak Qi flow to the Kidney Channel and the kidneys occurs between 5 and 7 p.m., and patients with kidney ailments may feel increased pain around 6 p.m.

Peak Qi flow to the Pericardium Channel occurs between 7 and 9

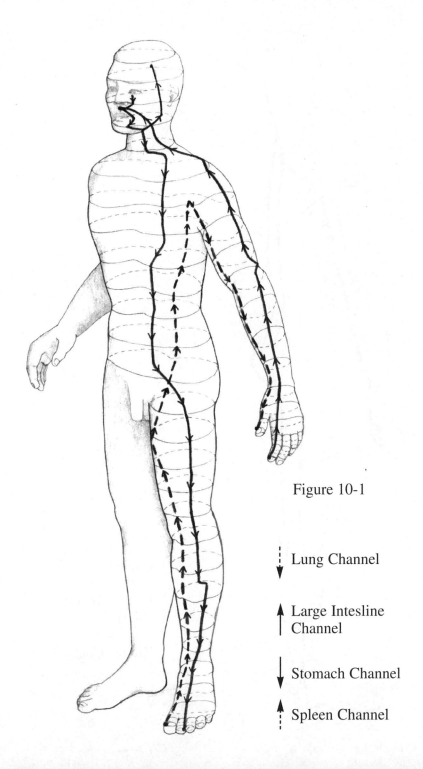

Figure 10-1

Lung Channel

Large Intesline Channel

Stomach Channel

Spleen Channel

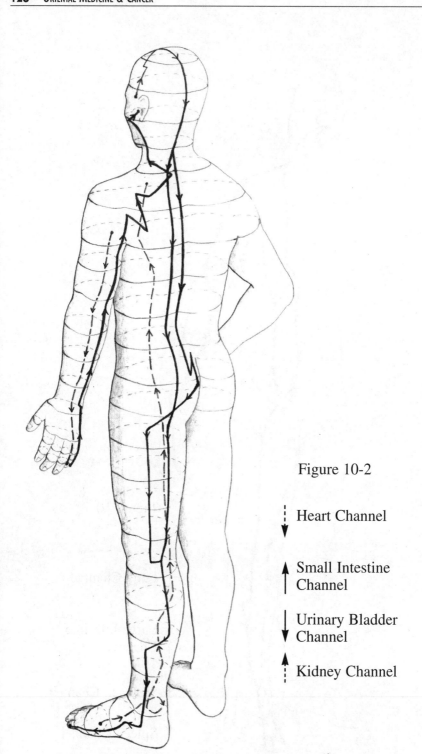

Figure 10-2

Heart Channel

Small Intestine
Channel

Urinary Bladder
Channel

Kidney Channel

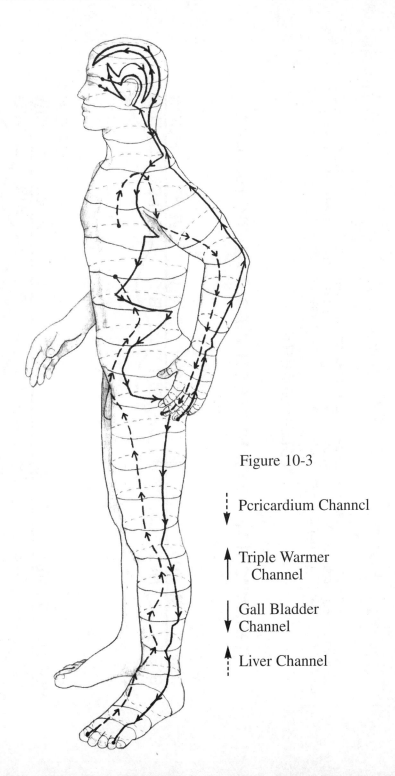

Figure 10-3

┊
▼ Pericardium Channel

▲
┃ Triple Warmer
     Channel

┃
▼ Gall Bladder
     Channel

▲
┊ Liver Channel

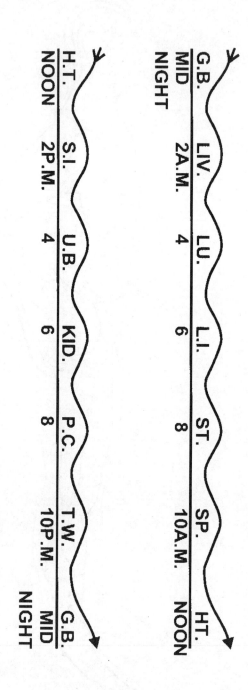

BIOLOGICAL QI CIRCULATION CLOCK OF EACH CHANNELS

G.B.	LIV.	LU.	L.I.	ST.	SP.	HT.
MID	2A.M.	4	6	8	10A.M.	NOON
NIGHT						

H.T.	S.I.	U.B.	KID.	P.C.	T.W.	G.B.
NOON	2P.M.	4	6	8	10P.M.	MID
						NIGHT

ABBREVIATION

LU. - LUNG	SP. - SPLEEN	U.B. - URINARY BLADDER
L.I. - LARGE INTESTINES	HT. - HEART	KID. - KIDNEY
ST. - STOMACH	S.I. - SMALL INTESTINES	P.C. - PERICARDIUM
		T.W. - TRIPLE WARMER
		G.B. - GALL BLADDER
		LIV. - LIVER

Figure 10-4

p.m., and patients with acute or epidemic high fever, as in malaria or encephalitis, will feel increased pain at 8 p.m. Experienced Western physicians have long known that patients with a febrile disease were likely to experience a sharp increase in body temperature between 7 and 10 p.m.

Peak Qi flow to the Triple Warmer Channel occurs between 9 and ll p.m., and there is increased likelihood of fever, ear ache or pain at 10 p.m.

Peak Qi flow to the Gall Bladder Channel and the gall bladder occurs between ll p.m. to l a.m., and liver disease patients may feel a mild fever which disturbs their sleep around midnight.

Peak Qi flow to the Liver Channel occurs between l a.m. and 3 a.m., and liver area pain is most likely to be felt around 2 a.m. These patients may experience disturbed sleep between midnight and 3 a.m.

There are still many Korean Taoist healers in the countryside and mountains who believe that a patient should be treated according to the channel time schedule. Thus asthma patients would be treated at either 4 a.m. or 4 p.m. (when the lung Qi flow is either at a maximum or minimum flow).

FIVE ELEMENT THEORY, YIN/YANG & THE THREE DIMENSIONAL MODEL

Over the last two thousand years, many scholars have attempted to understand what the relationship is between Five Element Theory and the Yin/Yang structure. The first chart included here, Figure 10-5, is the way in which this relationship is most commonly agreed upon by Chinese scholars.

Most people involved in Chinese medicine understand the Yin and Yang characteristics of the CV (Ren) and GV (Du) channels to be that the CV is the most Yin and the GV the most Yang channel on the body. From this it is easy to see what trigrams correspond to these two channels. The Quian trigram, with its three solid lines, corresponds to the GV Channel and the Kun trigram, with three broken lines, corresponds to the CV Channel. But the relationships between the other acupuncture channels and trigrams are not as easy to grasp.

Figures 6-6 to 6-11 show the development from a one dimension-

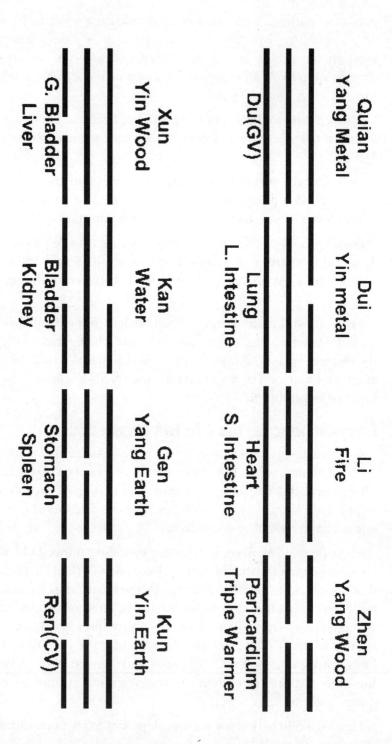

Figure 10-5

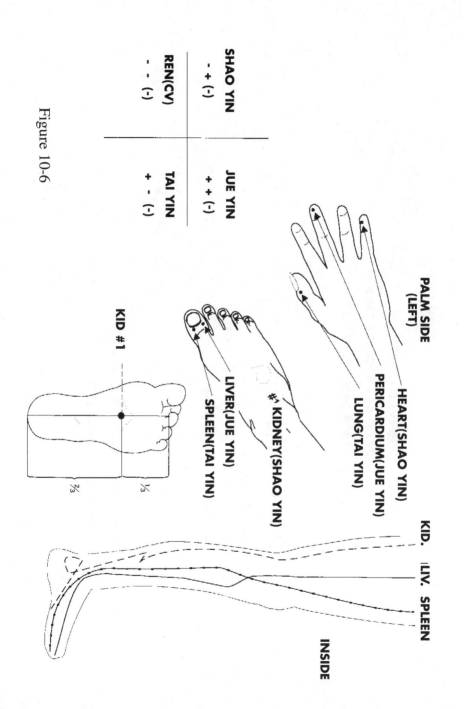

Figure 10-6

SHAO YIN	JUE YIN
- + (-)	+ + (-)
REN(CV)	TAI YIN
- - (-)	+ - (-)

PALM SIDE
(LEFT)

HEART(SHAO YIN)

PERICARDIUM(JUE YIN)

LUNG(TAI YIN)

LIVER(JUE YIN)

SPLEEN(TAI YIN)

#1 KIDNEY(SHAO YIN)

KID #1

⅔   ⅓

KID.   LIV.   SPLEEN

INSIDE

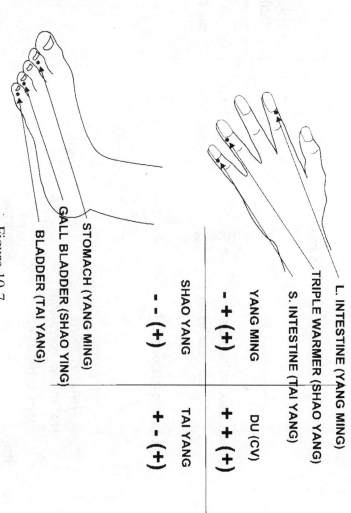

Figure 10-7

L. INTESTINE (YANG MING)

TRIPLE WARMER (SHAO YANG)

S. INTESTINE (TAI YANG)

	DU (CV)
YANG MING	
- + (+)	+ + (+)
SHAO YANG	TAI YANG
- - (+)	+ - (+)

STOMACH (YANG MING)

GALL BLADDER (SHAO YING)

BLADDER (TAI YANG)

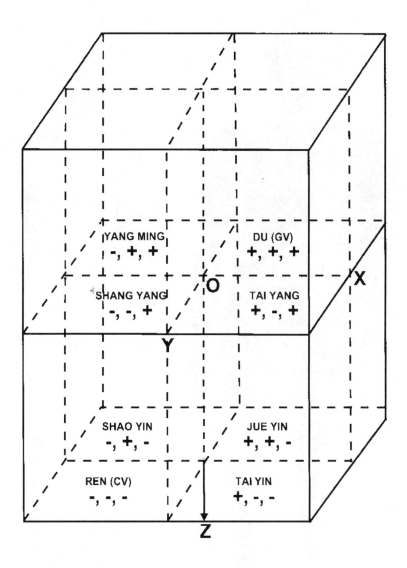

Figure 10-8

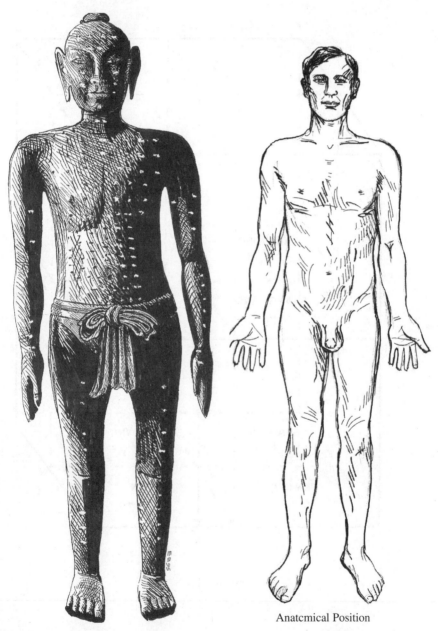

Figure 10-9

Anatcmical Position

Figure 10-10

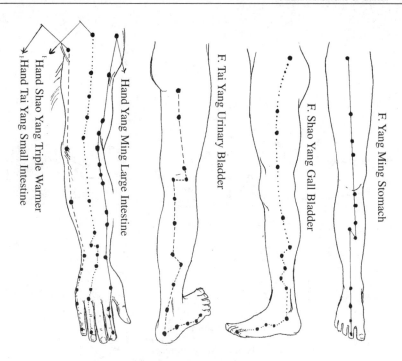

Hand Shao Yang Triple Warmer
Hand Tai Yang Small Intestine
Hand Yang Ming Large Intestine
F. Tai Yang Urinary Bladder
F. Shao Yang Gall Bladder
F. Yang Ming Stomach

Figure 10-11

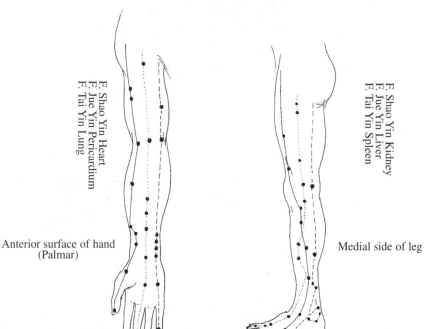

F. Shao Yin Heart
F. Jue Yin Pericardium
F. Tai Yin Lung

F. Shao Yin Kidney
F. Jue Yin Liver
F. Tai Yin Spleen

Anterior surface of hand
(Palmar)

Medial side of leg

Figure 10-12

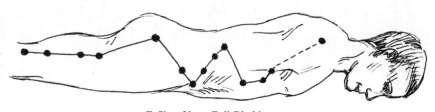

F. Shao Yang Gall Bladder

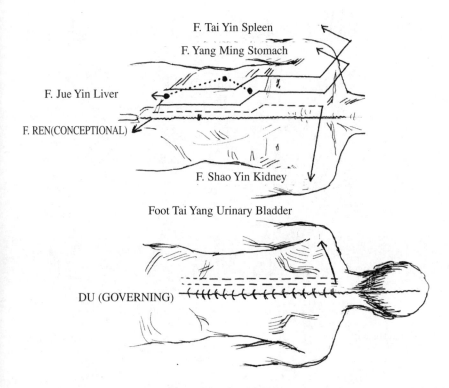

F. Tai Yin Spleen

F. Yang Ming Stomach

F. Jue Yin Liver

F. REN(CONCEPTIONAL)

F. Shao Yin Kidney

Foot Tai Yang Urinary Bladder

DU (GOVERNING)

Figure 10-13

al system to the three dimensional Cartesian coordinate system that I have developed. Figures 10-6 and 10-7 illustrate the application of this three dimensional system to the acupuncture channels themselves. From this it becomes easier to understand which of the trigrams corresponds to which channel. Figure 10-8 is a representation of the principle stated in the *Neijing* that the Yang channels circulate Qi through the surface of the body and the Yin channels circulate Qi through the interior of the body.

The acupuncture points depicted on the bronze statue appeared for the first time in Chinese history during the Song Dynasty (960-1279 A.D.). At that time the College of Chinese Medicine was established and had instituted a national licensing examination. Before the Song Dynasty the art of acupuncture had been handed down from father to son, from master to disciple in an apprenticeship system.

For the national licensing exam students had to insert needles correctly in holes in the bronze statue which had been filled with wax. Any candidate who failed the exam for two years was advised to find another profession. Figure 10-9 shows the bronze statue which was made during the Ming dynasty (1443 A.D.) and is still in existence in China as the oldest bronze acupuncture statue.

The question arises as to why this statue's palms face the sides of its body instead of forward as in the classic modern anatomic position (Figure 10-10). It is my feeling that the position of the hands is deliberate, perhaps as a teaching tool to point out the parallel configuration of the three hand and three foot channels:

Hand Yang Ming – Large Intestine   Foot Yang Ming – Stomach
Hand Shao Yang– Triple Warmer   Foot Shao Yang – Gall Bladder
Hand Tai Yang– Small Intestine   Foot Tai Yang – Urinary Bladder

Hand Shao Yin – Heart   Foot Shao Yin – Kidney
Hand Jue Yin – Pericardium   Foot Jue Yin – Liver
Hand Tai Yin – Lung   Foot Tai Yin – Spleen

Note: Yang Ming – Bright Yang   Jue Yin – Absolute Yin
         Shao Yang – Lesser Yang   Shao Yin – Lesser Yin
         Tai Yang – Greater Yang   Tai Yin – Greater Yin

The Hand Tai Yin Lung Channel, Hand Jue Yin Pericardium Channel, and Hand Shao Yin Heart Channel all flow on the palms and on the Yin side of the arms. They have the same spatial relationships to each other as the Foot Tai Yin Spleen Channel, Foot Jue Yin Liver Channel, and Foot Shao Yin Kidney Channel which flow through the Yin part of the leg, stomach and chest area, as Figure 10-12 illustrates.

If you compare the Yin and Yang paired channels (to be discussed in detail later in this chapter) which flow on the abdominal area on the side of the body and torso, the comparison is as follows (refer to Figure 10-13):

The Foot Tai Yang Urinary Bladder Channel flows beside the Du Channel (GV) on the back (Yang) side of the body and the Foot Shao Yin Kidney channel flows beside the Ren (CV) Channel on the front (Yin) side. The Foot Yang Ming Stomach Channel flows on the abdomen and chest between two Yin Channels, the Foot Shao Yin Kidney Channel and Foot Tai Yin Spleen Channel. The Foot Tai Yin Spleen Channel flows between two Yang Channels, the Foot Yang Ming Stomach Channel and Foot Shao Yang Gall Bladder Channel. The Foot Shao Yang Gall Bladder Channel flows between two Yang Channels, the Foot Yang Ming Stomach Channel and Foot Tai Yang Urinary Bladder Channel. The Foot Jue Yin Liver Channel flows between two Yin Channels, the Foot Tai Yin Spleen Channel and Foot Shao Yin Kidney Channel.

Some acupuncturists hypothesize on the subject of channel theory that the strongest Yang Qi flows through the Du (GV) Channel and the strongest Yin Qi flows through the Ren (CV) Channel. Therefore, since the Foot Tai Yang Urinary Bladder Channel is closer to the Du channel than the other two Yang Channels (Gall Bladder and Stomach), it would follow that more Yang Qi flows through the Urinary Bladder Channel than through the other two Yang Channels. They express this mathematically as :

Du > UB > GB > ST

Conversely when treating the Yin Channel flows, the mathematical expression is:

Ren > Kid > Liv > SP

However, it should be remembered that in one chapter of the *Yellow Emperor's Internal Medicine* the following advice appears. One should understand that the location of the Yin and Yang Channels indicate simply door and hinge. Don't think that their names indicate which channel has more Yin or Yang.

The channels can be categorized by the relative amounts of Qi and blood that flow through them as is shown in Figure 10-14. You will notice that not all the classical texts agree on the nature of the Yin channels, although there is unanimity regarding the Yang channels. This is probably due to mistakes made by manuscript copiers at some point in the past. In the days before photocopy machines books were copied by hand with ink and brush. Often this work was performed by people who were not knowledgeable scholars and mistakes were not uncommon. I choose to go along with the majority vote in cases where there are discrepancies, so I classify the Yin channels as follows:

Tai Yin-Abundant Blood, scanty Qi.

Jue Yin-Abundant Blood, scanty Qi.

Shao Yin-Scanty Blood, abundant Qi.

When the categories in Figure 10-15 are applied to the Qi following sequence of channels, the amount of Qi and Blood alternates between abundant and scanty in all cases except the Tai Yin-Yang Ming-Tai Yin sequence.

CHANNELS	CHAPTER 24 OF SU WEN	CHAPTER 65 OF LING SHU	CHAPTER 68 OF LING SHU
Tai Yang Small Intestine Urinary Bladder	Abundant Blood Scanty Qi	Abundant Blood Scanty Qi	Abundant Blood Scanty Qi
Shao Yang Triple Warmer Gall Bladder	Scanty Blood Abundant Qi	Scanty Blood Abundant Qi	Scanty Blood Abundant Qi
Yang Ming Large Intestine Stomach	Abundant Blood Abundant Qi	Abundant Blood Abundant Qi	Abundant Blood Abundant Qi
Tai Yin Lung Spleen	Scanty Blood Abundant Qi	Abundant Blood Scanty Qi	Abundant Blood Scanty Qi
Jue Yin Pericardium Liver	Abundant Blood Scanty Qi	Scanty Blood Abundant Qi	Abundant Blood Scanty Qi
Shao Yin Heart Kidney	Scanty Blood Abundant Qi	Abundant Blood Scanty Qi	Scanty Blood Abundant Qi

Fig. 10-14

TAI YIN	YANG MING	TAI YIN
Lung	Large Intestine/Stomach	Spleen
(ABUNDANT BLOOD – SCANTY QI) ⇐⟩	(ABUNDANT BLOOD – ABUNDANT QI)⇐⟩	(ABUNDANT BLOOD – SCANTY QI) ⇐⟩

SHAO YIN	TAI YANG	SHAO YIN
Heart	Small Intestine & Urinary Bladder	Kidney
(SCANTY BLOOD – ABUNDANT QI) ⇐⟩	(ABUNDANT BLOOD – SCANTY QI) ⇐⟩	(SCANTY BLOOD – ABUNDANT QI) ⇐⟩

JUE YIN	SHAO YANG	JUE YIN
Pericardium	Triple Warmer & Gall Bladder	Liver
(ABUNDANT BLOOD – SCANTY QI) ⇐⟩	(SCANTY BLOOD – ABUNDANT QI)⇐⟩	(ABUNDANT BLOOD – SCANTY QI) ⇐⟩

Fig. 10-15

CHANNEL PATHWAYS OF TRADITIONAL CHINESE MEDICINE

THE LUNG CHANNEL

The Lung Channel originates in the middle of the body and runs down internally to connect with the large intestine (A). It then turns upward, passing by the stomach (B) and through the diaphragm (C) before entering the lungs (D). From here, it rises to the throat and then emerges to the surface at Lu 1 under the clavicle. The Lung Channel runs externally down the medial aspect of the arm, passes by the radial artery at the wrist, and ends at the medial side of the tip of the thumb at Lu 11. A connecting channel runs from Lu 7 near the wrist (above the styloid process of the radius) to the radial side of the tip of the index finger, where it links to the Large Intestine Channel (see Figure 10-16).

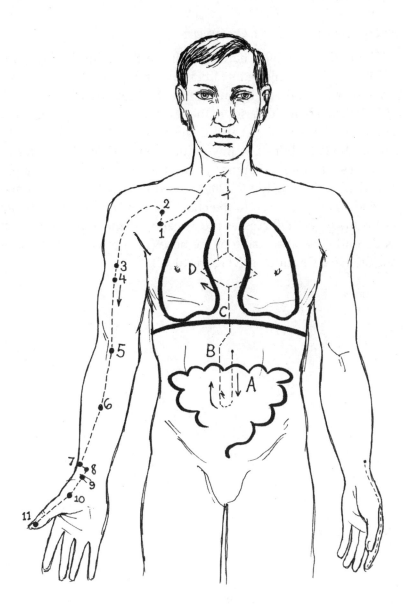

Hand Tai Yin
Lung Channel

Figure 10 -16

THE LARGE INTESTINE CHANNEL

The Large Intestine Channel begins at the tip of the index finger (LI 1) and runs up along its radial side. It then ascends along the lateral-anterior aspect of the arm to the highest point of the shoulder (LI 15). From here, it passes to the seventh cervical vertebra where it connects with Du 14 (A) and then crosses to the front of the body above the collarbone. At this point, the Channel divides into two branches. The internal branch connects downwards to the lungs (B), the diaphragm (C), and the large intestine (D). The external branch ascends along the neck to the cheek from where it enters the gums of the lower teeth. It crosses the upper lip to the opposite side of the body and ends at the side of the nose (LI 20), where it connects to the Stomach Channel (see Figure 10-17).

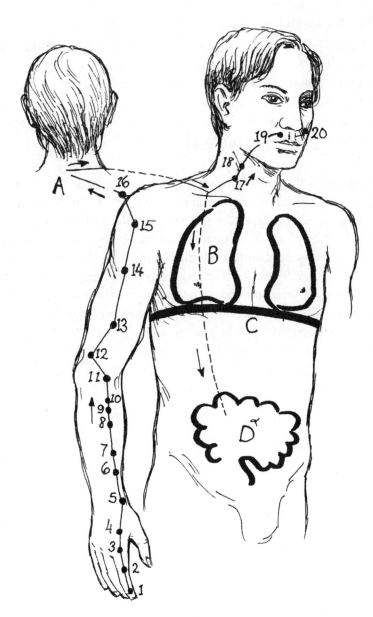

Hand Yang Ming
Large Intestine Channel

Figure 10 -17

THE STOMACH CHANNEL

The Stomach Channel begins internally at the side of the nose. It ascends the bridge of the nose and connects with the Urinary Bladder Channel at the inner corner of the eye (UB 1). It emerges below the eyeball (St 1) and then descends, entering the upper gums and curving around the lips. From under the mouth it follows the lower jaw, then turning upward passes in front of the ear to the forehead.

From St 5 the channel runs down along the throat to the area above the collarbone. An internal branch descends from there through the diaphragm (A), entering the stomach (B), and connecting with the spleen (C). The external branch runs downward along the chest, passing through the nipple and past the umbilicus to the groin (St 30). At this point it reconnects with the internal channel. From here, the channel descends the front of the leg all the way to the lateral side of the second toe. There are two branches below the knee. One runs from just below the knee (St 36) to the lateral side of the middle toe. The second leaves from the top of the foot (St 42) and connects to the Spleen Channel at the medial side of the big toe (see Figure 10-18).

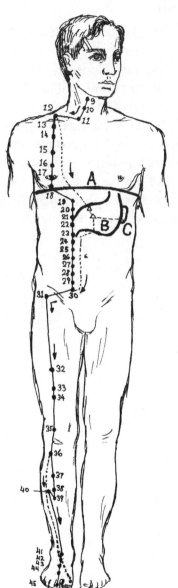

Foot Yang Ming
Stomach Channel

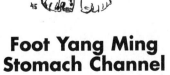

Figure 10 -18

THE SPLEEN CHANNEL

The Spleen Channel begins on the inside of the big toe (Sp 1) and runs along the inside of the foot, turning upwards in front of the inner ankle. It then ascends along the inside of the leg to the abdomen. At Sp 15, lateral to the umbilicus, an internal pathway connects with the spleen (A) and the stomach (B) and then runs up through the diaphragm (C) to the heart (D), where the Spleen and Heart Channels connect. The main channel continues to ascend to the chest, and from Sp 20 another internal pathway runs upward through the throat and terminates on the lower surface of the tongue. The main channel descends from Sp 20 and ends at Sp 21 on the side of the rib cage (see Figure 10-19).

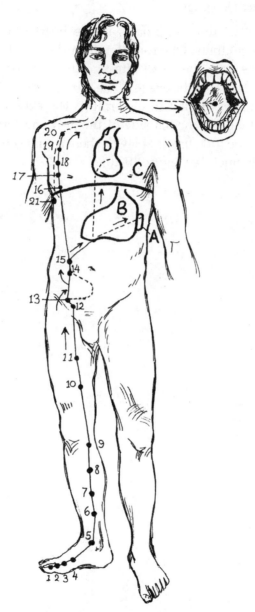

Foot Tai Yin
Spleen Channel

Figure 10 -19

THE HEART CHANNEL

The Heart Channel originates in the heart (A). Three internal branches begin there. One runs downward through the diaphragm and connects with the small intestine (B). A second runs upward through the throat to the eye (C). The third passes through the lungs (D) and emerges at Ht 1 in the armpit. The external channel then descends along the medial side of the arm and terminates on the inside tip of the little finger at Ht 9, where it connects with the Small Intestine Channel (see Figure 10-20).

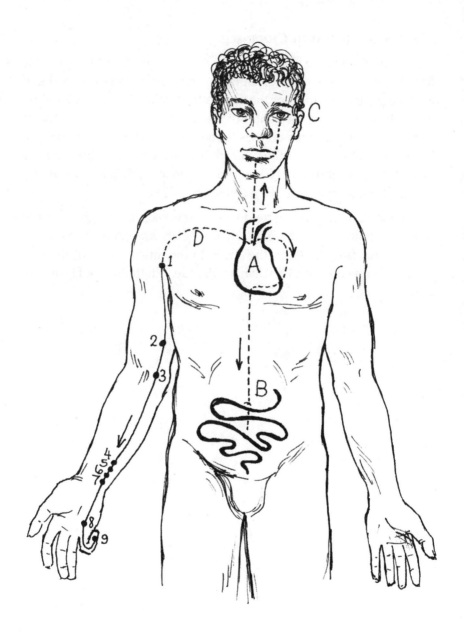

Hand Shao Yin
Heart Channel

Figure 10 -20

The Small Intestine Channel

The Small Intestine Channel begins on the outside of the tip of the little finger at SI 1. It ascends along the inside of the back of the hand and the posterior aspect of the arm to the back of the shoulder joint. From there it runs to the center of the upper back where it connects with Du 14 (A) and then crosses to the front of the body. An internal branch separates above the collar bone and descends through the heart (B), the diaphragm (C), and the stomach (D), before terminating at the small intestine (E) (see Figure 10-21).

The external channel ascends along the neck to the cheek, from where it connects to the ear, where the channel ends at SI 19. A branch runs from SI 18 on the cheek to the inner corner of the eye, where it connects with the Urinary Bladder Channel (see Figure 10-21).

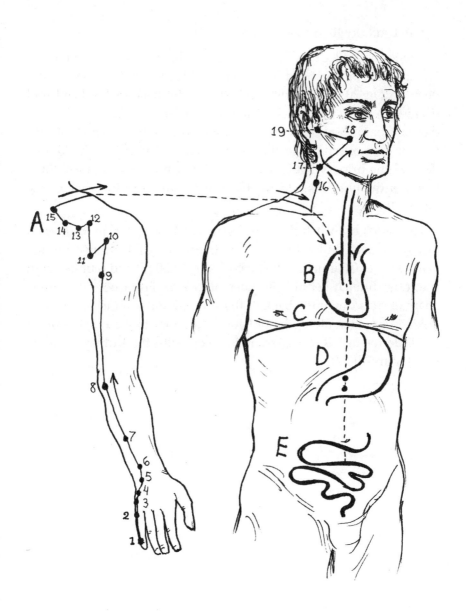

Hand Tai Yang
Small Intestine Channel

Figure 10 -21

THE URINARY BLADDER CHANNEL

The Urinary Bladder Channel starts at the inner corner of the eye and ascends the forehead to the vertex of the head (A), where it connects to Du 20. It then descends along the back of the head and divides in two at the back of the neck. Both branches continue to descend parallel to the spine. The inner branch has an internal connection that originates in the lumbar region and enters the kidney (B) and the urinary bladder (C). The inner branch continues down through the buttocks and the back of the thigh to the back of the knee (D).

The outer branch follows the same course as the inner branch down the back, but is further from the spine (E). It connects to the Gall Bladder Channel on the buttocks at GB 30 (F) and reunites with the inner branch behind the knee at UB 40. From here the single channel runs down the back of the calf (G) and around the outside ankle bone, then along the outside of the foot to the outside tip of the little toe at UB 67, where it connects with the Kidney Channel (see Figure 10-22).

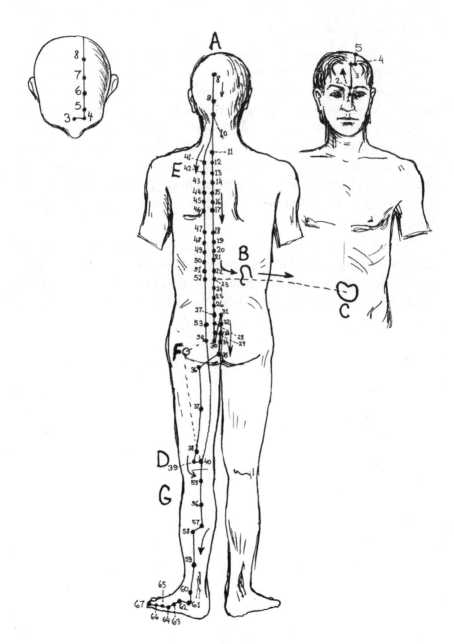

Foot Tai Yang
Urinary Bladder Channel

Figure 10 -22

The Kidney Channel

The Kidney Channel starts on the underside of the little toe and runs along the sole of the foot (K 1). From there it runs under the navicular bone and behind the inner ankle. Then it ascends the inner side of the leg to the top of the thigh (A). An internal branch runs from here to the base of the spine (A) where it connects to Du 1. The internal branch then ascends along the lumbar spine and enters the kidney (B) and the urinary bladder (C). Another internal branch runs from the kidney up to the liver (D), the diaphragm (E), the lung (F), and continues through the throat to the base of the tongue (G).

The main channel ascends from the inner thigh up the abdomen and the chest to the collarbone where it ends at K 27. From the lung, a branch joins the heart and flows into the chest where it connects with the Pericardium Channel (see Figure 10-23).

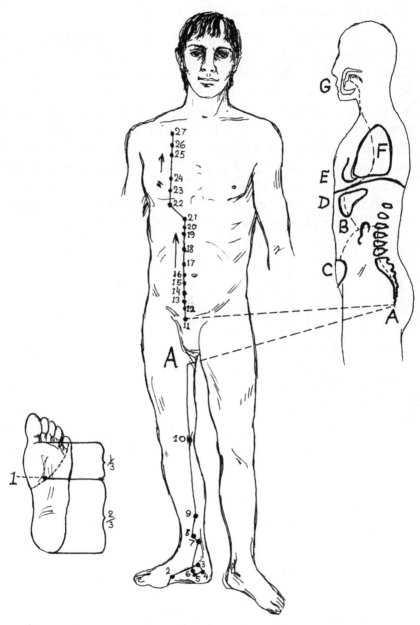

Foot Shao Yin
Kidney Channel

Figure 10 -23

The Pericardium Channel

The Pericardium Channel originates in the chest and enters the pericardium (A). An internal branch descends through the diaphragm (B) to the abdomen (C), connecting with the Upper, Middle, and Lower portions of the Triple Warmer. Another internal branch runs from the middle of the chest to an area just lateral to the nipple where it emerges at P 1. The external channel runs from here through the armpit and then down the medial aspect of the arm all the way to the palm of the hand at P 8. From this point the main channel extends to the tip of the middle finger where it ends at P 9. A branch runs to the tip of the ring finger, where it connects with the Triple Warmer Channel (see Figure 10-24).

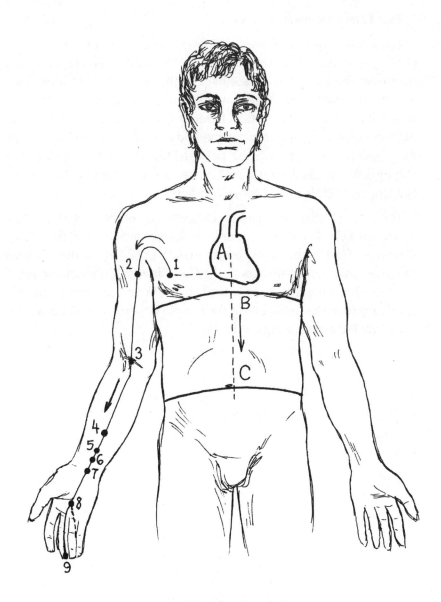

Hand Jue Yin
Pericardium Channel

Figure 10 -24

THE TRIPLE WARMER CHANNEL

The Triple Warmer Channel originates at the tip of the ring finger (TW 1) and runs between the fourth and fifth metacarpal bones, then over the wrist and up the back of the arm to the shoulder joint at TW 14. From here it goes across the back of the shoulder (A) where it connects with the Gall Bladder Channel at GB 21. The channel then crosses to the front of the body. An internal branch enters the chest to connect with the pericardium (B) and then descends through the diaphragm (C) and down to the abdomen (D), linking the Upper, Middle, and Lower Warmers.

The external channel ascends along the side of the neck to the base of the ear (TW 17), from where it circles behind the ear, then turns downward to the cheek and terminates at TW 23 at the outer corner of the eye, where it connects to the Gall Bladder Channel. An internal branch on the face runs from TW 20 above the ear up onto the head and then descends along the temple before connecting with SI 18 below the eye (see Figure 10-25).

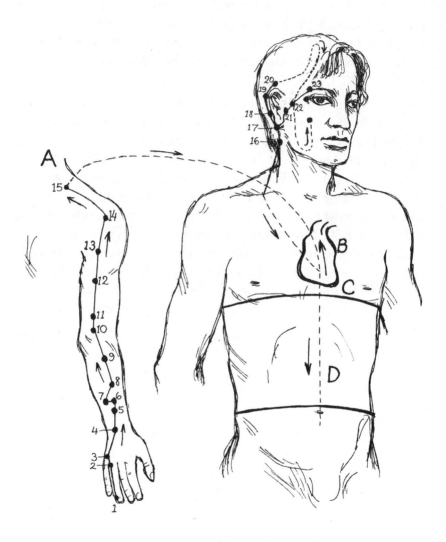

Hand Shao Yang
Triple Warmer Channel

Figure 10 -25

THE GALLBLADDER CHANNEL

The Gall Bladder Channel begins at the outer corner of the eye at GB 1. From here an internal branch descends through the neck and the chest through the diaphragm to the liver (A) and the gall bladder (B). It then continues downward along the side of the abdomen and connects with the main channel on the side of the buttock (C) at GB 30.

The external channel ascends to the corner of the forehead (GB 4), circles behind the ear (GB 12), then returns to the forehead (GB 14), before descending to the back of the neck and the top of the shoulder (GB 21). An internal branch runs from here to the back, connecting with Du 14, UB 11, and SI 12. From the top of the shoulder the main channel descends (D) in front of the armpit and along the side of the chest and torso to the hip where it intersects the internal branch at GB 30. The single channel then descends along the outside of the leg, passes in front of the outer ankle and over the back of the foot before ending at GB 44 on the outside of the fourth toe. From GB 41 on the back of the foot, a branch crosses over to the big toe, where it connects with the Liver Channel (see Figure 10-26).

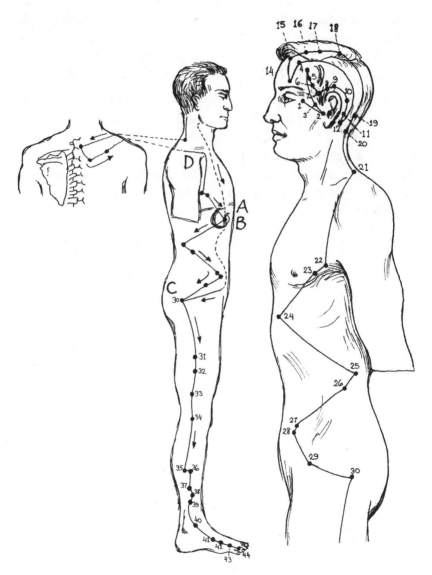

Foot Shao Yang
Gall Bladder Channel

Figure 10 -26

The Liver Channel

The Liver Channel begins on the top of the big toe and runs upward along the back of the foot to the front of the inside ankle. It then ascends the inside of the leg until it reaches the genital region. After encircling the genitals it runs up the abdomen until it reaches LIV 13 below the rib cage, where an internal branch separates. The main external channel then terminates at LIV 14 below the nipple.

The internal branch enters the liver (A) and connects with the gall bladder (B). It then ascends, crossing the diaphragm (C) and entering the lungs (D) where it connects with the Lung Channel and completes the cycle. An internal branch continues upwards from here through the throat to the eye (E) and then up to the vertex of the head. Another branch descends from the eye to encircle the mouth (see Figure 10-27).

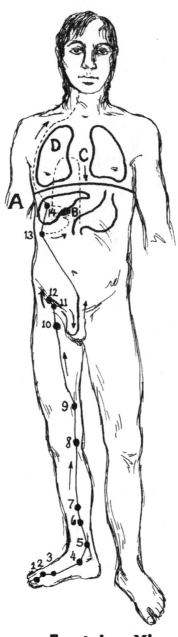
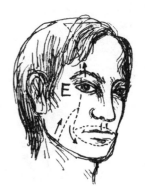

Foot Jue Yin
Liver Channel

Figure 10 -27

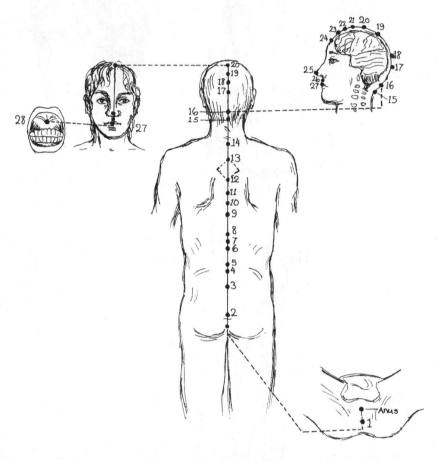

GV
DU Channel

Fig. 10 -28

THE DU (GV) CHANNEL

The Du Channel begins in the lower abdomen and descends internally to emerge at Du 1 between the anus and the coccyx. It then ascends the midline of the back and the head to the vertex (Du 20) from where it descends across the forehead and the tip of the nose before ending at Du 28 inside the upper lip (see Figure 10-28).

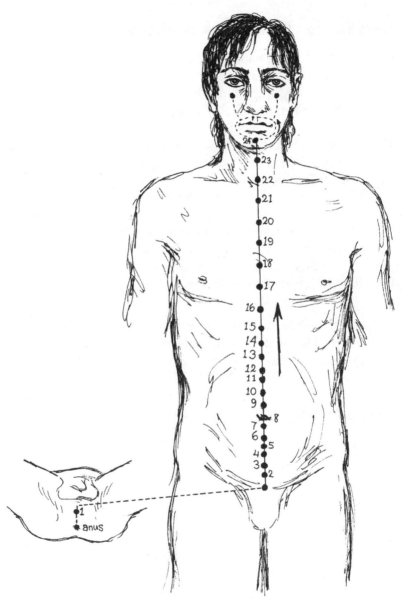

Fig. 10 -29

THE REN (CV) CHANNEL

The Ren Channel begins in the lower abdomen and descends internally before emerging at REN 1 between the anus and the genitals. It then ascends along the midline of the abdomen and chest before ending at REN 24 below the lower lip. Internal pathways from this point encircle the lips and extend upwards to St 1 just below the eyes (see Figure 10-29).

Myung Kim's Three Dimensional Four Inter-Channel Theory

Hand Tai Yin Lung Channel (4 a.m.)
    Hand Yang Ming L. I. Channel (6 a.m.)
    Foot Yang Ming Stomach Channel (8 a.m.)
Foot Tai Yin Spleen Channel (l0 a.m.)

Hand Shao Yin Heart Channel (l2 Noon)
    Hand Tai Yang S. I. Channel (2 p.m.)
    Foot Tai Yang U. B. Channel (4 p.m.)
Foot Shao Yin Kidney Channel (6 p.m.)

Hand Jue Yin Pericardium Channel (8 p.m.)
    Hand Shao Yang Triple Warmer Channel (l0 p.m.)
    Foot Shao Yang Gall Bladder Channel (12 Midnight)
Foot Jue Yin Liver Channel (2 a.m.)

As you can see from the above chart, four channels make one set and any problem with an internal organ and/or channel can affect the other related channels and organs (refer to Figures 10-1, 10-2, 10-3).

(1) Hand Yin/Yang Paired Channel Theory

    A) Hand Tai Yin Lung Channel
       Hand Yang Ming Large Intestine Channel

    B) Hand Shao Yin Heart Channel
       Hand Tai Yang Small Intestine Channel

    C) Hand Jue Yin Pericardium Channel
       Hand Shao Yang Triple Warmer Channel

Note for above chart:

The Yin and Yang channel relationships for a, b, and c above are as follows:

The Large Intestine Channel supplies Qi to the lung. This can be through LI16.

The Small Intestine Channel supplies Qi to the heart. This can be through SI11.

The Triple Warmer Channel supplies Qi to the pericardium. This can be through TW15.

(A) HAND TAI YIN LUNG CHANNEL

Hand Yang Ming Large Intestine Channel <Metal>

A problem of the lung or Lung Channel will disturb the Qi flow of the Large Intestine Channel and will affect the nose function. As a general rule of thumb, treat chronic lung problems through the Lung Channel. Treat acute problems, such as cough, sneezing or allergy attacks through the Large Intestine Channel primarily. LI16 is used as a Qi supplying point to the lung.

(B) HAND SHAO YIN HEART CHANNEL

Hand Tai Yang Small Intestine Channel <Fire>

Problems of the heart or Heart Channel will disturb the Qi flow of the scapula area and through the neck and ear where the Small Intestine Channel passes. If a patient's left side H3 point is more tender than the right, SI 11 on the same side in the middle of the scapula will likewise be tender. Also the patient will experience ear problems and hear strange noises.

For a patient with chronic heart problems, treat the Heart Channel. If the heart problem is acute, primarily treat acupuncture points on the Small Intestine Channel. SI 11 is used as a Qi supplying point to the heart.

(C) HAND JUE YIN PERICARDIUM CHANNEL

Hand Shao Yang Triple Warmer Channel <Fire>

If a patient contracts an epidemic disease causing high fever, the pericardium and the Pericardium Channel will be affected and the Triple Warmer Channel will affect the ear causing ear pain and ear infection.

If a patient has a chronic pericardium problem, then treat

acupuncture points on the Pericardium Channel. However, if a patient develops an acute pericardium problem, such as a high fever, then treat primarily the acupuncture points on the Triple Warmer Channel. Triple Warmer 15 on the back is the best point to supply Qi to the pericardium and to control a high fever.

(2) BROTHER CHANNEL THEORY

A) Hand Yang Ming Large Intestine Channel
   Foot Yang Ming Stomach Channel

B) Hand Tai Yang Small Intestine Channel
   Foot Tai Yang Urinary Bladder Channel

C) Hand Shao Yang Triple Warmer Channel
   Foot Shao Yang Gall Bladder Channel

(A) HAND YANG MING LARGE INTESTINE CHANNEL

Foot Yang Ming Stomach Channel.

The pathways of these two channels are identical in relationship to the hand, arm, foot and leg. They meet beside the nose (LI 20) and under the eye (ST 1). They can be considered as one channel because the Large Intestine Channel starts at the tip of the second finger and ends at the tip of the second toe of the Stomach Channel. When one point of the Large Intestine Channel is stimulated by acupuncture, its Qi will travel via the Stomach Channel and supply Qi to the Large Intestine.

Now let us consider LI 10 (Shou San Li- Hand Three Mile) and ST 36 (Zu San Li - Foot Three Mile). Their names are identical; their proportional distances from the elbow and knee are the same; their treatment indications are similar. The problems of one organ or one channel will affect the other organ or the other channel. If one is injured at the ankle area (ST 41), then the Qi flow of LI 5 (Thumb side of the wrist area) will be disturbed. A knee joint injury at ST 35 will affect the elbow joint LI11 area. If a person is injured anywhere between the clavicle area and the second toe of the stomach channel, this injury will affect ST 12 (just above the clavicle) and LI 15 (the front part of the shoulder) and this will disturb Qi flow to the entire

Large Intestine Channel. Likewise the Qi flow disturbance can originate in the Large Intestine Channel and then affect the Stomach Channel.

(B) HAND TAI YANG SMALL INTESTINE CHANNEL

Foot Tai Yang Urinary Bladder Channel

The pathways of these two channels are identical in relationship to the hand, wrist, foot and ankle. They meet at Ear (SI19) and Eye (UB 1 area). They can be considered as one channel because the Small Intestine Channel starts at the tip of the small finger and the Urinary Bladder Channel ends at the tip of the small toe. When one point of the Small Intestine Channel is stimulated by acupuncture, its Qi will travel via the Urinary Bladder Channel and supply Qi to the small intestine. Problems of one channel or its respective organ will affect the other channel or its organ.

If a person injures the cervical vertebrae or neck area, it will affect the area between UB11 and SI 15 on the upper back and disturb Qi flow to the entire Small Intestine Channel. Acupuncture points around the scapula area such as SI 14, 13, 12, 11, 10 and 9 will show stiffness and soreness. The Qi flow of the heart will also be disturbed and pain and numbness will radiate down to the small finger. Likewise the problem can originate in the Small Intestine Channel and progress to the Urinary Bladder Channel.

(C) HAND SHAO YANG TRIPLE WARMER CHANNEL

Foot Shao Yang Gall Bladder Channel.

The pathways of these two channels are identical in relationship to the hand, arm, foot and leg. They meet at the end of the eyebrow (TW 23) and near the lateral end of the eye (GB 1). They can be considered as one channel because the Triple Warmer Channel starts at the tip of the 4th (ring) finger and the Gall Bladder Channel ends at the tip of the 4th toe. When one point of the Triple Warmer Channel is stimulated by acupuncture, its Qi will travel via the Gall Bladder Channel and supply Qi to the Triple Warmer. The problems of one channel or its organ will affect the other channel or its organ.

If a person has pains at GB 40 (ankle area straight above the fourth toe), that person will experience pains at TW 4 (wrist area). A pain at GB 33 (2 or 3 inches above the knee joint) will show pains at TW 11 (elbow area). Pains at GB 21 (halfway between the 7th cervical vertebra and the end of the shoulder) will travel to TW 15 and will have an effect through TW 1 at the tip of the fourth (ring) finger. Likewise the problem can originate in the Triple Warmer Channel and proceed to the Gall Bladder Channel.

(3) Foot Yin/Yang Paired Channel Theory

A) Foot Yang Ming Stomach Channel
   Foot Tai Yin Spleen Channel <Earth>

B) Foot Tai Yang Urinary Bladder Channel
   Foot Shao Yin Kidney Channel <Water>

C) Foot Shao Yang Gall Bladder Channel
   Foot Jue Yin Liver Channel <Wood>

(a) Foot Yang Ming Stomach Channel

Foot Tai Yin Spleen Channel <Earth>

Problems of digestion are related to the Stomach and Spleen Channels. The pathways of these two channels are very close to each other on the leg and stomach area. Qi can be supplied directly to the lung, large intestine, stomach, and spleen through the Stomach Channel. The two organs are considered as the element Earth according to the Five Element Theory, and problems in either one of the channels will affect the other. For chronic problems of digestion, treat primarily the Spleen Channel. For acute problems of digestion, treat primarily the Stomach Channel.

(b) Foot Tai Yang Urinary Bladder Channel

Foot Shao Yin Kidney Channel <Water>

The relationship between the urinary bladder and the kidney is easily understandable. Blood and water are filtered by the kidney, and urine flows through the urinary bladder. Qi can be supplied directly to the heart, the small intestine, the urinary bladder and the kidney through the Urinary Bladder Channel. Both the kidney and the urinary bladder are considered as the element Water according to the Five Element Theory, and a problem in either channel will affect the other. Any pain between UB11 and 30 (neck area to hip area on both sides of the spine) will evidence itself between K11 and K27 (lower abdominal area to below the clavicle near the center line of the body). For chronic kidney problems, treat primarily the Kidney Channel. For acute kidney problems, treat primarily the Urinary Bladder Channel.

(c) Foot Shao Yang Gall Bladder Channel

Foot Jue Yin Liver Channel <Wood>

The relationship between these two channels is as close as the proximity of their organs would naturally indicate. Qi can be supplied directly to the pericardium, triple warmer, gall bladder and liver through the Gall Bladder Channel. The two organs are considered as the element Wood in the Five Element Theory and a problem in either channel will affect the other. I will explain these channels in more detail in a later chapter of this book. For chronic liver problems, treat primarily the Liver Channel. For more acute liver problems, treat primarily the Gall Bladder Channel.

(4) Sister Channel Theory

A) Hand Tai Yin Lung Channel
    Foot Tai Yin Spleen Channel

B) Hand Shao Yin Heart Channel
    Foot Shao Yin Kidney Channel

C) Hand Jue Yin Pericardium Channel
    Foot Jue Yin Liver Channel

(A) Hand Tai Yin Lung Channel

Foot Tai Yin Spleen Channel

One example illustrating the relationship of these two channels is expressed by the following: "Damp phlegm invades the lung."

If a person consumed only vegetables, salad or cold foods for a prolonged period for dietary reasons and/or if the weather were damp and cold, damp phlegm can be formed. In acute cases the phlegm will invade the lung, but in chronic cases, it will invade the spleen. Symptoms of damp in the Lungs are shortness of breath, coughing up watery phlegm and initial signs of asthma. Acute symptoms are shortness of breath when lying down and stuffiness in the chest. On the surface of the tongue a dirty, greasy-looking coat can form. A patient with heat will show a yellow coat; one with cold will show a white coat. In this case the pulse will be slippery like that of a woman pregnant for six months. Symptoms of damp in the Spleen include lethargy, nausea, vomiting, and a heavy feeling in the head as though it were wrapped up in a towel. Sometimes people with low blood pressure exhibit similar symptoms.

(B) Hand Shao Yin Heart Channel

Foot Shao Yin Kidney Channel

"Communication between the Heart and Kidney"

According to the Five Element Theory the Kidney is considered to be the element Water and the Heart to be the element Fire. A problem in either organ or channel can affect the other organ or channel. In modern hospitals it is observed that patients with kidney disease are likely to get heart problems, and, likewise, patients with heart disease are likely to acquire kidney complications. Some patients have both heart and kidney disease simultaneously.

"Heart Fire"

When emotional stress, anxiety and/or anger accumulate, Qi stasis can result. Then explosions of Liver Fire can become Heart Fire. Symptoms include dry throat, headache, darkening color of urine and sometimes hematuria (blood in urine). The face and body can become hot and sleep may be disturbed. These symptoms are explained in the language of Oriental Medicine as "Heart Fire moving through the Small Intestine Channel and then affecting the Urinary Bladder and the Kidney Channel."

(C) HAND JUE YIN PERICARDIUM CHANNEL

Foot Jue Yin Liver Channel

Both channels are related to heat or fever in the body. Acute feverish disease can disturb the Qi flow to the ear and cause ear pain and infection via the Triple Warmer Channel. The Gall Bladder Channel and the Liver Channel can also be affected.

Emotional stress can cause internal heat in the Liver Channel resulting in "Liver Qi stagnation." As expressed in Oriental Medicine, "Liver Yang rising" and "Liver Fire" gradually affect the Gall Bladder Channel, the Triple Warmer Channel and the Pericardium Channel. This can cause Qi stagnation, mild heat, and anger, rather than acute fever. I'll explain these symptoms in the Chapter 11, which follows.

CHANNEL THEORY & PERSONAL CHARACTERISTICS

It is very difficult to isolate a single emotional trait out of the complex interactions that make up the human psyche. But I believe that it is possible to place people in broad categories. For example, some people are born with introspective and quiet personalities (Yin) and others with outgoing, aggressive personalities (Yang). Someone born with a congenital Lung weakness will have a tendency towards sadness and melancholy, while someone with a Kidney weakness will be more fearful.

This should not be seen as a substitute for an understanding of psychological factors which originate in someone's environment or family upbringing. Obviously personal experiences have a tremendous impact on how someone looks at the world. But consider differing emotional responses within a single family. Imagine that one member of a large family is killed by a drunken driver. Family members will react to this tragedy in different ways. Some will be more sad and others more angry. Someone could be so mad that he or she wants to kill the drunken driver and someone else's reaction could be a life-long depression. Perhaps Oriental Medicine can help to explain these widely varying reactions to a single event. Some responses will be acute and some chronic, some excess and some deficient, some more Yin and some more Yang in nature. And some may correspond to the emotions associated with the different organs in Five Element Theory.

I have found that there are three major groups of emotions, which after the application of Yin/Yang theory break down into six types of people. Of course just as with Yin and Yang there are no pure emotional characteristics but psyches that are changing and that often contain elements of more than one type, but each person does have predominant characteristics that place him or her in one group or another.

GROUP 1

| Tai Yin | Lung/Spleen |
| Yang Ming | Large Intestine/Stomach |

People in this category are dominated by sadness and worry. They are sensitive and think too much and will often display lung and digestive problems. Their Qi moves slowly and tends to stagnate all over the body.

GROUP 2

| Shao Yin | Heart/Kidney |
| Tai Yang | Small Intestine/Urinary Bladder |

People in this category are fearful and easily frightened. As I described in the Heart section of Chapter 12, all the Shen, Ling, Hun, and Po points are located in the Heart, Kidney, and Urinary Bladder Channels. The Qi of people in this category usually stagnates in the lower parts of their body.

GROUP 3

| Jue Yin | Pericardium/Liver |
| Shao Yang | Triple Warmer/Gall Bladder |

People in this category are dominated by anger and irritability. Generally their Qi rises excessively to their head.

CHANNEL THEORY & DISEASE PATTERNS

Someone's body constitution, disease and injury history, and life style can cause different types of channel problems. For example:

Someone who catches cold easily and has digestive problems will have

| Tai Yin | Lung/Spleen |
| Yang Ming | Large Intestine/Stomach |

Someone who does not get enough exercise and consumes too much fat is likely to have Heart and Kidney weakness and will have:

| Shao Yin | Heart/Kidney |
| Tai Yang | Small Intestine/Urinary Bladder |

Someone under a lot of mental stress or susceptible to anger and/or someone with lower back problems will have

| Jue Yin | Pericardium/Liver |
| Shao Yang | Triple Warmer/Gall Bladder |

Many people actually have multiple channel problems due to inherited weak organ functions, bodily injuries, and/or emotional trauma. In my practice I find that my Asian patients most often display Tai Yin/Yang Ming problems. The second most common group is Shao Yin/Tai Yang, and Jue Yin/Shao Yang is the rarest.

Western males display a somewhat similar distribution, with Tai Yin/Yang Ming again the most common, but Jue Yin/Shao Yang second and Shao Yin/Tai Yang the least often seen. Western women have a very different pattern of channel problems. I most often see Jue Yin/Shao Yang, Shao Yin/Tai Yang is second and Tai Yin/Yang Ming the rarest. Western women tend to participate in sports more often than Asian women do and recent medical studies have indicated that women who participate in sports have a greater frequency of knee injuries than men. I suspect that this is because women have wider hips which places greater stress on the knee. This would also explain the greater occurrence of Shao Yang channel problems and back injuries among Western women.

If you consider your own personal constitution, your history of bodily injuries and your mental stress level using the criteria I have presented here, you should be able to come up with some ideas regarding your own disease patterns and prognosis.

QI IFUSION

When giving Qi to a patient, most patients will be able to see colors when they close their eyes. If any of the following colors are bright it means that the Qi flow is better and the prognosis is better than if the color is darker (see Figure 10-30).

Interpretation of colors

- Red – Fever, excessive anger
- Blue – Stress, Qi or Blood Stagnation
- Green – Liver Qi stagnation or Gall Bladder channel pain
- Yellow – Stomach or digestive problems
- White – Lung weakness
- Dark – Qi Deficiency

Rainbow or diamond color - Best prognosis. Most often seen by younger people or those who practice Zen meditation.

How much Qi a patient can feel during the course of a treatment depends upon the strength of his or her constitution and the ability of the practitioner. In many cases, a patient can feel tingling sensations or a warm feeling radiating through the body when an acupuncturist places Qi into the body through a needle. If a patient suffers severe Qi stagnation and Qi deficiency that is caused by chronic illness, surgery, an accident, or old age the patient might not feel any Qi sensation at all during the initial treatment. As the recovery progresses with subsequent treatments, however, the patient will feel more Qi sensation during each visit.

More detailed information about giving Qi to a patient will be provided in my upcoming book on Qi Gong.

Proper use and exercise of the fingers will stimulate the acupuncture channels there, but overuse and abuse will cause blockages of Qi to develop in those channels. This can lead to carpal tunnel syndrome. Japanese finger massage (Shiatsu) practitioners can develop thumb problems because of overuse of the thumb in their practice. Because the Lung channel passes through the thumb, Qi can become stagnated there and eventually a Lung Qi Deficiency problem can result.

In Japanese gangster (Yakuza) movies you will sometimes notice characters who have had the small finger on their left hand cut off as a gang punishment. Probably such a person will develop heart trouble later in life as the Heart channel passes through the little finger.

The losses of other parts of the body will have different effects. The loss of a toe or toes in an accident will have an effect on the channel that passes through that toe and eventually the function of the organ itself will be weakened. A polio victim or someone who has had a leg amputated will suffer different problems depending upon which side is lost. If the left, probably the heart and spleen will be affected and if the right is lost more likely the liver and gall bladder functions will be impaired. I am basing this upon the location of the organ in the body, but thorough surveys need to be done to determine the actual effects.

Sometimes after acupuncture treatment when patients begin to regain strength in their arms or especially in their legs, they over-exercise or walk too great a distance, which can again make their problem worse. Also at times a physical therapist will put too much stress on a newly-strengthened arm or leg and make it worse again. It is important for the acupuncturist to caution the patient. When the Qi flow is stimulated it will enable more blood and sensations of warmth to travel through the affected arm or leg and it can feel markedly better very quickly. However it may be months before the muscle is truly strong enough for even mild physical exercise. In the meantime, counsel the patient to use moxa, warm water treatment, herbal medicine, and Qi Gong exercise as indicated and not to be in a hurry.

Conversely even patients with very serious problems of paralysis or polio should not give up even when they do not feel that they are getting any better. Continuing to get acupuncture and herbal treatments and massage and staying with the home moxa and hot water treatments and Qi Gong practice can help even in very difficult

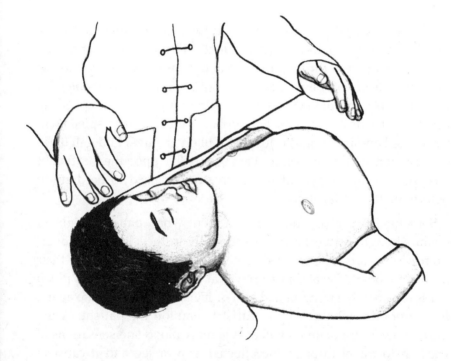

Qi Infusion

Figure 10 -30

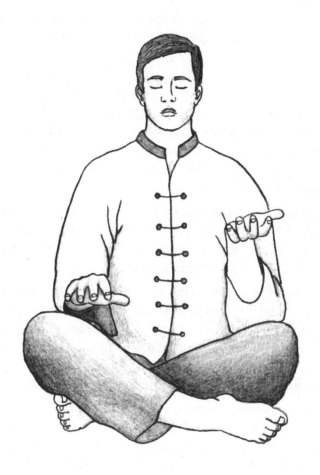

**Absorb Qi from Heaven and EARTH
One of the Buddhist Style Qi Gong Positions**

Figure 10 -31

cases.

MODERN ACUPUNCTURE

Some Chinese practitioners continue to use long needles, 2-3 inches in length or even longer. But most acupuncturists in America today use hair-thin (0.2 mm) needles with insertion tubes for rapid insertion and no sensation of pain. Also most use disposable needles because of the potential spread of infectious diseases like hepatitis or HIV. Of course it is possible to sterilize needles just like doctors and dentists sterilize their equipment, but to do so requires the use of an autoclave run at 250° Fahrenheit (121° C) for 30 minutes. Precision is essential to insure sterility and most acupuncturists just find disposable needles preferable.

Ear acupuncture has become very popular since its systematization by Paul Nogier. Points are needled during treatment and also small (3 mm) intradermal needles are used which the patient can wear for 3-5 days between treatments.

Electro-acupuncture is widely used for acute pain, sports injuries, and chronic joint pain. Machines running on either AC current or 9 volt DC batteries can produce a variety of frequencies of vibration producing strong or mild stimulation. Heart patients with pacemakers should not be given electro-acupuncture. Extreme caution should be used if running current across the chest with anyone.

I check the patient by touching both sides of the body with a needle to compare the degree of sensation on each side. Someone with polio, a stroke or long-term channel blockage will have different sensations on each side. An interesting finding that I have made is that even in milder case of channel blockage when needles are inserted bilaterally and stimulated with electricity much more stimulation is required on the blocked side to feel sensation equal to that on the normal side.

CASE STUDY

Abby K. was a 30 year-old woman who had had breast reduction surgery on both sides and 3-inch horizontal scars under her breasts. She also suffered from a left side Gall Bladder channel blockage which resulted from a lower lumbar vertebrae injury. When I used electro-acupuncture on her I set the Gaze control to 3 on her right side, a level at which she felt a good level of stimulation. But on her left side even at level 6 she felt nothing. I was forced to go as high as 8 before she felt a sensation equal to the right side. Each patient will feel different degrees of sensation and never assume that what is right for one will be right for another. This is because everyone's Qi flow and channel stagnation situation is different.

I recommend electro-acupuncture for the treatment of surgery scars, especially on the abdomen. It will not only open up Qi flow to the affected channel but also cause the scars to flatten as is done with cosmetic surgery. I will write in more detail on my findings with scar treatment in future professional seminars.

There is an unorthodox style of bee sting acupuncture which has been influenced by German homeopathic medicine. In Europe they have found that giving people bee stings in their fingers has cured arthritis. Of course some people are allergic to bee stings and for them a treatment like this can be very dangerous. This treatment is not legal in the U.S., but I know that it is being used by some Asian Americans in California and Caucasians in New England.

EMERGENCY TREATMENT

If you find someone in an emergency situation, the steps you take could save a life. I believe that everyone should have first aid training to be prepared to help in an emergency and this section is not meant as a substitute for such training. But there are additional steps that someone can take if they know what to do that I am going to outline here as well as reminding you of some first aid basics.

Before even calling 911, you should first be sure that the scene is safe and then check the victim's condition. It is important to be calm, to talk and walk slowly and softly, and to comfort the victim verbally as Western first aid training advises. Do not move a seriously injured victim unless there is an immediate danger. The first thing to check is whether or not the person is conscious. If not, call for an ambulance at once! Now you need to check to see whether or not the victim is breathing and perform rescue breathing if they are not and you are trained to do so.

What if the person is conscious but the face is very pale and the person is feeling faint? You can immerse the hands and feet in warm water to stimulate Qi circulation. If you are outdoors or somewhere where warm water is not available you can rub the hands and feet vigorously with your hands and warm them that way.

If the person has a high fever and his or her eyes are beginning to roll back so that more of the white is showing, you can pierce the person's finger tips next to the nail beds with a lancet or a needle. Or just puncture the tip of the middle finger. All you want to do is make a small hole so that you can squeeze out a few drops of blood and allow some of the heat to escape.

If the condition is more severe and the high fever is accompanied by tremors or delirium or the person begins to lose consciousness you can also puncture Du 26, the point located at the center of the upper lip below the nose. If you don't have an acupuncture needle handy press the point hard with your thumb. At the same time place your other hand on top of the person's head so that the center of your palm rests on Du 20, the point at the vertex. Once the person's consciousness is stable, cover him or her with a blanket and keep as comfortable as possible.

Traditional Chinese medicine teaches that Kidney 1 on the sole of the foot and Pericardium 8 at the center of the palm can also be needled in an emergency situation. I feel that both for psychological and sanitary reasons these points should be avoided. If a patient is very weak, the pain of needling these points may be enough to send him or her into shock.

I believe that the warm water technique is the most useful for a wide range of emergency situations including:

- fainting
- severe psychological or emotional imbalances such as extreme anger, sadness, fear
- dizziness
- nausea
- heart attack
- severe bleeding. First stop the bleeding and then apply the warm water technique.

• heat stroke or high fever. First puncture the finger tips as describe above and then immerse the feet in warm water for 2 minutes. Afterwards immerse the hands in warm water.

If someone is suffering from stomach cramps or indigestion, never warm up the stomach area. This will only make the pain worse. Instead use the warm water technique on the hands and feet. Then have the patient lie on his or her stomach and give a vigorous finger massage to the UB 21 area. (This is the Stomach Back Shu point located 1.5 cun [37] lateral to the lower border of the twelfth thoracic vertebra.) This may cause the patient to feel a sharp pain just above the waist line. Then have the patient turn on the back and apply moxa or rub with your hands to warm up the following points around the navel: Stomach 25 (2 cun lateral to the center of the navel on both sides) and REN 12 (on the midline of the abdomen 4 cun above the navel).

Muscle cramps can also be relieved by the warm water treatment. Muscle cramps are Yin in nature, so they need to be treated with Yang energy which can be supplied by rubbing the cramped muscle. But it is much more effective to use warm water to stimulate the flow of blood and circulation of Qi as I have already described. I was watching the Atlanta Olympics this summer when the young American swimmer was stricken with muscle cramps. As she lay by the side of the pool in agony, her trainers tried to massage away the cramps. I wanted to shout at them through the television to just place her hands and feet in warm water. Her discomfort would have been eased much sooner.

MYUNG KIM'S ACUPUNCTURE POINT PALPATION DIAGNOSTIC METHOD

First, check the patient's pulse and examine the tongue as is done in Traditional Chinese Medicine (TCM). After this, press SI 8, H 3, and LI 11, all of which are located at the patient's elbow. Also check TW 4 at the wrist and H 9 on the small finger. For these last two points, press with the dull end of a toothpick. What you are trying to do here is to compare the sensations of each point on the left and right sides. You will find that most people have more tender Heart points on the left side because two thirds of our heart is located on the left side of our body. After this, press REN (CV) 17 and a few Ah Shi points between this point and the nipples. (Ah Shi points are areas other than acupuncture points that are pain sensitive when pressed with a finger.) Usually, the patient will complain that the left side is more sensitive than the right.

After this, have the patient lie on a table in a prone position to check the back. In China, Korea, and Japan the back is generally ignored during the diagnostic process. Historically in Asia the focus was on digestive problems and chronic diseases and the emphasis was on examining the abdomen. But today in the West we treat many more musculo/skeletal problems and physical injuries. So I place a lot of emphasis on examining the back when I diagnose a patient.

Begin with the Back Shu points along the Bladder channel that correspond to the organs which had the weakest pulses. Also check the lumbar area and if the patient complains of pain or sensitivity there inquire about sciatic pain and also press UB 40 and UB 60. You should also ask about muscle cramps and palpate the hamstring area between UB 36 and 37 (Semitendinosus and/or biceps femoris muscles) and the calf (gastrocnemius muscle) between UB 57 and 58. Ask the patient about knee weakness and whether the patient hears cracking sounds, especially when climbing stairs. While the patient is lying in this position also press Kid 1 on the sole of the foot. If there are kidney problems, the more painful foot will indicate which kidney is involved.

In the case of a woman, you also need to inquire about ovary pain. If she suffers from this, it is important to know whether it occurs only before menstruation or whether it is always present with varying degrees of intensity.

Next move to GB 30 and the Reproduction Point (see Kim's acupuncture points) for Gall Bladder channel problems. You will find that many people are sensitive in this area. Also check the neck area. Do not take your patient's word that the neck is fine. Lots of people have minor discomfort that they are so accustomed to that they forget about it. So take the time to palpate each cervical vertebra thoroughly with your finger tips. If you do find discomfort anywhere in the neck, press SI 9 and SI 11 and the Small Intestine Extra Point.

If the patient has demonstrated Gall Bladder channel problems that manifest more on the left side check SI 11, UB 15 (Heart Shu point), and UB 20 (Spleen Shu point) looking for signs of a Heart and Spleen Qi Deficiency. If there has been more pain on the right side then check UB 18 and 19, the Liver and Gall Bladder Shu points respectively.

In general, a problem on one side of the body will affect either the neck or lower back on the same side. This occurs because the flow of Qi is disturbed on the injured side and that will eventually affect the spine on that same side. The exception to this can occur when someone is involved in a car accident. I have seen patients who have a lower back problem on the left side and a neck problem on the right and vice versa, but this type of case is rare.

A UB/Tai Yang channel problem in the lower back can manifest directly as a SI/Tai Yang channel problem or through a same side neck problem. A GB/Shao Yang channel problem can manifest as a TW/Shao Yang channel problem as well. Check TW 14 and 15 for sensitivity and if the patient complains of problems like ear ache or infection or vertigo then check TW 17 just below and behind the ear.

Having done all the above, it is time to ask the patient to turn over and lie in a supine position. The first step is to check the Front Mu points corresponding to whichever organs showed pathological problems according to your TCM pulse diagnosis.

Next move to the Gall Bladder Channel. If a patient's ankle (GB 40 area) is painful there will probably be more pain on that same side of the body. Check GB 31 on the thigh. Now bend the knees up so that the soles of the feet are flat on the floor. This will relax the abdominal muscles, allowing you to check GB 28 for potential hernia problems or a tilted uterus, if the patient is a woman.

For women, GB 22 and 23 as well as Pericardium 1 and Spleen 18, all of which are located on the lateral side of the nipple, are points to check for future breast tumor problems. Stomach 16 and 18, directly above and below the nipple can also be checked. Liver 8-12 are all important to examine for gynecological problems as well. Ask the male patient to squeeze both testes to find out which side is smaller or more painful. As you have done while examining the back, if you have found right side GB Channel problems use them to guide you to the appropriate side of the body. Be sure to palpate

LIV 14 and GB 24 on the right side. Both of these points lie on a line extending down from the nipple. If there is a sharp pain at LIV14 or at GB24 (both are located under the nipple), then there is a possibility of liver or gall bladder problems or gall stones.

Observation of the patient is also important. For example, someone may have one eye which is smaller than the other, the line between the nose and the corner of the mouth may be deeper on one side, or a patient might complain of more varicose veins on one side than the other. These are probably due to Gall Bladder, Urinary Bladder, and Stomach channel problems which have persisted on that affected side for many years.

Always be sure to look for surgery or accident scars. These can cause blockages of Qi flow in any channels that they cut across. Ask the patient what the scar was caused by. Sometimes a scar may appear vertical on the outside of the body but actually be the result of a horizontal incision on the inside. This is particularly the case with Caesarean sections and other abdominal operations. And you need to know where the inside incision took place when you are considering what channels may be blocked.

Another diagnostic method utilizes a wooden pole that is between 1 1/2 and 2 inches in diameter and at least 2 feet long. Ask the patient to hold the pole horizontally with their thumbs underneath and to squeeze it forcefully. They may notice a weakness or blockage along one of the channels of the arm when they do this. As the patient is squeezing the pole, you can also pull it away from their body and have them try to tug it back. This may make it easier for them to notice where the channel weakness or blockage is located.

CARPAL TUNNEL SYNDROME

An Example of Myung Kim's Diagnostic Method

Carpal tunnel syndrome is usually associated in peoples' minds with typists or computer programmers who perform the same motions over and over again while holding their hands in an awkward position. But it can also result from heavier work like landscaping or construction. Someone who uses a jackhammer can damage the nerves in the wrists from the continuous pounding that he or she is subjected to. This nerve damage can even affect the dilation and construction of blood vessels in the hands when they are subjected to changes in temperature. This can even lead to frostbite in the hands in more extreme cases.

1. Ask the patient which hand and wrist are more painful.

2. Check for any surgical or injury scars that cross acupuncture channels, especially on the hand or arm.

3. Does the patient suffer from arthritis of the shoulder, elbow, or fingers?

4. Is there any history of wrist or elbow injury? If so, are there problems with the knee or ankle on the same side. Be sure to check the GB 40 (ankle) and TW 4 relationship.

5. Check the cervical vertebrae of the neck and whether problems there are reflected on the Small Intestine channel between SI 8 at the elbow and SI 9 on the back of the shoulder. Don't forget the Small Intestine Extra Point!

6. Check the Gall Bladder channel and whether any problems there have radiated to the Triple Warmer channel. If so Triple Warmer 11 near the elbow and 14 and 15 on the shoulder will probably be sensitive.

7. Check Stomach 35 on the lateral side of the knee joint and the extra point Xiyan on the medial side. Problems here usually come from Gall Bladder channel problems and often the elbow on the same side will also be affected. If this becomes chronic, eventually the Large Intestine channel will also be affected. Pulled muscles or tendons, pinched nerves, and sprained elbow joints will all be more likely to happen on the same side as the knee problem.

8. Usually carpal tunnel syndrome begins on the Yang side of the arm, especially along the Small Intestine and Triple Warmer channels. Later the Large Intestine channel and the three Yin channels of the arm (Heart, Pericardium, and Lung) can become involved. Most commonly, pain will radiate along the Pericardium channel, which passes through the carpal tunnel at the pathway of the median nerve.

9. You will probably end up treating carpal tunnel syndrome via

the following channels:

Bladder to Small Intestine - Tai Yang foot to Tai Yang arm channel (Brother)

Gall Bladder to Triple Warmer - Shao Yang foot to Shao Yang arm channel (Brother)

Stomach to Large Intestine - Yang Ming foot to Yang Ming arm channel (Brother)

Triple Warmer to Pericardium - Shao Yang arm to Jue Yin arm channel (Yin/Yang Pair)

Liver to Pericardium - Jue Yin foot to Jue Yin arm channel (Sister)

Hair Treatment

I am presenting here my approach to the treatment of baldness and hair loss as one example of how Oriental Medicine is applied differently to each individual, even those who appear to suffer from the identical condition. I am sure it will also be of interest to any readers who are suffering from these problems themselves to know that they can be helped.

Hair is an indicator of the total health of our body. I have identified seven different conditions that can have a negative impact on the health of the hair. Some of these conditions can exist simultaneously in the same individual, as hair loss is due to both emotional stress and physical problems.

1. Severe mental stress can block the flow of Qi in the Gall Bladder Channel through Liver Qi Stagnation. In Korea, children as young as ten years of age can begin to show bald patches on their heads. These children tend to be the ones who are forced to go to school all day and then study additional subjects like music, martial arts, computers, and foreign languages outside of school so that they can get ahead.

2. Yin Deficiency can be a cause, especially for post-menopausal women. The dryness that accompanies Yin Deficiency can affect their skin, eyes, and hair. The internal organs can also become drier, resulting in constipation.

3. A condition of dryness in the Lungs, or other lung-related problems like exposure to cigarette smoke or air pollution can cause

dry skin and hair according to Oriental medical theory. A fifty year-old woman came to my office suffering from hair loss and a skin problem (psoriasis). She had a history of bronchitis and had had contracted pneumonia many times since childhood, so it was obvious that she had a constitutional Lung weakness. Recently she had also lost one of her younger sons in a car accident, and the grief and sadness she was experiencing had further affected her Lungs, as these are the emotions associated with the Lungs in Five Element Theory.

4. Another cause can be a Deficiency of Kidney Qi and Kidney Jing. This is most commonly seen in people over seventy, but some young people who have chronic illnesses show this kind of pattern as well. In severe cases not only does their hair fall out but even their teeth can become loose.

5. Physical injuries and scars on the acupuncture channels, especially the Urinary Bladder, Gall Bladder, Triple Warmer, and Stomach, can interrupt the flow of Qi in these channels. This can cause loss of hair where these channels cross the scalp. If the flow is blocked on the left side GB Channel, the hair loss will be seen on the part of the head where the GB Channel runs on the left side and so on.

6. Hair loss can also result from severe dermatitis or burns. This type is very difficult to treat with acupuncture.

7. Inheritance is another factor. Some people have prematurely gray hair or baldness which they have inherited from their parents or grandparents. This does not necessarily mean that they have inherited a "hair problem gene." It can also indicate that they have inherited a tendency to become stressed too easily, or inherited a tendency toward a destructive lifestyle, such as alcoholism.

CASE STUDY

A fifty-five year-old Asian woman came to my office complaining of hair loss. Upon examination I found that she had a menopausal Yin Deficiency syndrome. I felt that she needed herbal medicine to tonify her Yin more than she needed acupuncture, but she had an American husband and thought that he might object to the smell of an herbal decoction, so she did not want to take herbs. I therefore offered her an herbal Yin tonic in pill form. She took this for a few days but felt that it was causing her stomach discomfort and wanted to stop. I insisted that she keep taking it for a while and that her stomach problems would improve, but she gave up taking the pills. Every time she came for a visit she would tell me that she doubted that acupuncture would really be able to improve her hair problem. In addition to her Yin Deficiency she had lower back pain associated with Gall Bladder Channel Qi blockage and a neck problem due to the blockage of Qi flow in the Bladder and Small Intestine Channels. I treated these problems as I normally would, but it felt as though her resistance made it difficult for me to make my Qi flow smoothly. After ten treatments she gave it all up without any improvement.

Why include a case study that does not have a successful outcome? You should always keep in mind if you receive treatment from a Doctor of Oriental Medicine, or a Western physician for that matter, that it is important to have a positive and cooperative attitude towards your doctor. This will facilitate the flow of Qi through your body and the doctor's as well. In the case of the patient that I have described here, her attitude may have contributed to the lack of improvement in her hair condition. And the fact that the treatments opened the blockages in her GB, SI, and UB Channels and may have prevented many possible bad consequences in her future is something that she will never be aware of.

Each individual has his or her own individual factor or combination of factors that may cause a hair loss problem. There are many possible treatments that may be effective. One should try massage and moxa on acupuncture points, meditation, and Qi Gong exercise. Herbal medicines and acupuncture treatments can make even transplanted hair grow thicker and healthier. The important thing is to try and not to give up hope.

Suggested points for massage and moxa treatment:

Lung 2 and 7

Gall Bladder 20, 21, and 40

Triple Warmer 4 and 17

Du (Governor Vessel) 20

Large Intestine 4

Liver 3

Spleen 6

Kidney 3

Urinary Bladder 60

Heart 7

Or also try points on other channels that correspond to the individual patient's organ disharmony or physical injury.

I CHING • THE BOOK OF CHANGES

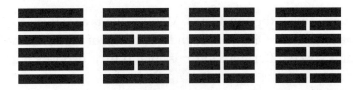

Figure 10 -32

The *I Ching* has been used in China for thousands of years. For most people, two trigrams are combined and the resulting hexagrams have been used to study the past and present situations of a person, a family, or even a nation as well as to predict the future. Today its use is still popular among many Asian fortune tellers for these purposes. Every Taoist will have a different opinion on the use of this classic work and the correct interpretation of the eight trigrams and sixty four hexagrams that make up the *I Ching*.

As I wrote in Chapter 6 (Yin/Yang Theory) I look at the eight trigrams as a three dimensional model of reality. The three additional lines of the hexagrams represent additional dimensions where time and space have natures that are beyond the perception of ordinary people (see Figure 10-32). Acupuncture itself can be described using this theory.

0. Point - In geometry, a point indicates a location but does not occupy an area. Acupuncture at its simplest level looks only at points.

1. Line - A one dimensional entity. A slightly more advanced acupuncturist understands the use of a channel to connect points in order to diagnose and treat disease.

2. Plane - A two dimensional figure. An acupuncturist working at this level is able to use relationships between two channels in his or her practice.

3. Space - The three dimensions in which we perceive the world. An accomplished acupuncturist understands and utilizes the relationships between all the channels in his or her practice.

4. Qi - At this level it becomes possible to understand the flow of Qi in the universe. Time and space are understood differently than by the ordinary person who perceives them only in three dimensions.

5. Shen - This is the spirit level. Many patients are affected on this level as well as the Qi level. An understanding of this level and how time and space differ makes it possible to treat people's Shen disturbances properly.

6. Ling – This is the level of the spirits of the dead. It is also the level at which prayer works, where one can receive guidance from entities like Buddha or Jesus. People do become possessed by spirits and they can be helped both with acupuncture and by appeals to the Ling spirits of their ancestors or benevolent Ling spirits variously described as Taoist immortals, the Holy Spirit, and so on.

POINTS FOR QI TONIFICATION AND GENERAL HEALTH IMPROVEMENT

LIV 3

SP 6

UB 23

GB 21

ST 36

CV 6

H 3

LI 4

CV 12

TO STIMULATE LABOR

Moxa and massage

Sp 6

UB 60

UB 67 - 30 minutes of moxa to turn breach birth

UB 26 - Both sides of 5th lumbar vertebra

Liv 8

Liv 3

UB 24 - Both sides of 3rd lumbar vertebra

UB 31 - Both upper sacral foramen.

Often the 4th lumbar vertebra is punctured to remove spinal fluid for diagnosis or to inject an anesthetic solution. But after the delivery of the baby many women suffer from lower back and sciatic pain affecting the Urinary Bladder and sometimes the Gall Bladder channel.

THE LUO (CONNECTING) POINTS OF THE YIN/YANG PAIRED CHANNELS OF TCM

Lung Channel	LI 6
Large Intestine Channel	LU 7
Stomach Channel	SP 4
Spleen Channel	ST 40
Heart Channel	SI 7
Small Intestine Channel	H 5
Urinary Bladder Channel	K 4
Kidney Channel	UB 58
Pericardium Channel	TW 5
Triple Warmer Channel	P 6
Gall Bladder Channel	LIV 5
Liver Channel	GB 37

Treat these points when one channel problem starts affecting Yin/Yang Paired Channel.

Back Shu points usually correspond to acute disease symptoms and Front Mu points are more often used to treat chronic disease. These points are also used for palpation diagnosis and as treatment points for many of the fundamental acupuncture treatments in TCM.

	BACK SHU	FRONT MU		BACK SHU	FRONT MU
LUNG	UB 13	Lu 1	URINARY BLADDER	UB 28	REN 3
LARGE INTESTINE	UB 25	St 25	KIDNEY	UB 23	GB 25
STOMACH	UB 21	Ren 12	PERICARDIUM	UB 14	REN 17
SPLEEN	UB 20	Liv 13	TRIPLE WARMER	UB 22	REN 5
HEART	UB 15	Ren 14	GALL BLADDER	UB 19	GB 24
SMALL INTESTINE	UB 27	REN 4	LIVER	UB 18	Liv 14

LOCATIONS OF THE BACK SHU & FRONT MU POINTS

BACK SHU POINTS

UB 13 (Feishu)   1.5 cun lateral to the midline of the back, at the level of the lower border of the spinous process of the third thoracic vertebra.

UB 14 (Jueyinshu)   1.5 cun lateral to the midline, at the level of the lower border of the spinous process of the fourth thoracic vertebra.

UB 15 (Xinshu)   1.5 cun lateral to the midline, at the level of the lower border of the spinous process of the fifth thoracic vertebra.

UB 18 (Ganshu)   1.5 cun lateral to the midline, at the level of the lower border of the spinous process of the ninth thoracic vertebra.

UB 19 (Danshu)   1.5 cun lateral to the midline, at the level of the lower border of the spinous process of the tenth thoracic vertebra.

UB 20 (Pishu)   1.5 cun lateral to the midline, at the level of the lower border of the spinous process of the eleventh thoracic vertebra.

UB 21 (Weishu)   1.5 cun lateral to the midline, at the level of the lower border of the spinous process of the twelfth thoracic vertebra.

UB 22 (Sanjiaoshu) 1.5 cun lateral to the midline, at the level of the lower border of the spinous process of the first lumbar vertebra.

UB 23 (Shenshu)   1.5 cun lateral to the midline, at the level of the lower border of the spinous process of the second lumbar vertebra.

UB 25 (Dachangshu)   1.5 cun lateral to the midline, at the level of the lower border of the spinous process of the fourth lumbar vertebra.

UB 27 (Xiaochangshu)   1.5 cun lateral to the midline, at the level of the first posterior sacral foramen.

UB 28 (Pangguangshu)   1.5 cun lateral to the midline, at the level of the second posterior sacral foramen.

FRONT MU POINTS

GB 24 (Riyue)   Directly below the nipple in the seventh intercostal space.

GB 25 (Jingmen)   On the lower border of the free end of the twelfth rib.

Liv 13 (Zhangmen) Below the free end of the eleventh rib.

Liv 14 (Qimen)   Directly below the nipple in the sixth intercostal space.

Lu 1 (Zhongfu)   At the lateral side of the first intercostal space, 6 cun lateral to the Ren Channel.

Ren 3 (Zhongji)   On the midline of the abdomen, 4 cun below the umbilicus.

Ren 4 (Guanyan)   On the midline 3 cun below the umbilicus.

Ren 5 (Shimen)   On the midline 2 cun below the umbilicus.

Ren 12 (Zhongwan) On the midline 4 cun above the umbilicus.

Ren 14 (Juque)   On the midline 6 cun above the umbilicus.

Ren 17 (Tanzhong) On the midline level with the fourth intercostal space, midway between the nipples.

St 25 (Tianshu)   2 cun lateral to the center of the umbilicus.

LOCATION OF THE SPIRIT POINTS

UB 15 - Xin Shu   Heart's Hollow - 1.5 cun lateral to the fifth thoracic vertebra.

Ren 14 - Ju Que   Great Palace - On the midline of the abdomen, 6 cun above the umbilicus.

Ren 8 - Shen Que   Spirit's Palace - In the center of the umbilicus.

Du 10 - Ling Tai   Spirit's Platform - Below the spinous process of the sixth thoracic vertebra.

Du 11 - Shen Dao   Spirit's Path - Below the spinous process of the fifth thoracic vertebra.

Du 24 - Shen Ting   Spirit's Hall - 0.5 cun directly above the midpoint of the anterior hairline.

UB 44 - Shen Dang Spirit's House - 3 cun lateral to the fifth thoracic vertebra, on the spinal border of the scapula.

H 7 - Shen Men   Spirit's Gate - At the ulnar end of the transverse crease of the wrist, in the depression on the radial side of the flexor carpi ulnaris tendon.

K 23 - Shen Feng   Spirit's Seal - 2 cun lateral to the Ren Channel in the fourth intercostal space.

K 25 - Shen Cang   Spirit's Storage - 2 cun lateral to the Ren Channel in the second intercostal space.

UB 42 - Pohu   Soul's Household - 3 cun lateral to the third thoracic vertebra, on the spinal border of the scapula.

UB 47 - Hunmen   Soul's Door - 3 cun lateral to the ninth thoracic vertebra.

H 4 - Ling Dao   Spirit's Path - On the radial side of the flexor carpi ulnaris tendon, 1.5 cun above the transverse wrist crease.

K 24 - Ling Xu   Spirit's Ruins - 2 cun lateral to the Ren Channel in the third intercostal space.

Location of the 13 Ghost Points

Du 26 (Ghost Palace)   A little above the midpoint of the philtrum, near the nostrils.

Lu 11 (Ghost Convincing) On the radial side of the thumb, about 0.1 cun posterior to the corner of the nail.

Sp 1 (Ghost Fortress)   On the medial side of the big toe, 0.1 cun posterior to the corner of the nail.

Lu 9 (Ghost Heart) At the radial end of the transverse crease of the wrist, in the depression on the lateral side of the radial artery.

UB 62 (Ghost Road) In the depression directly below the external malleolus.

Du 14 (Ghost Pillow)   Below the spinous process of the seventh cervical vertebra.

Du 16 (Ghost Bed) 1 cun directly above the midpoint of the posterior hairline, directly below the external occipital protuberance, in the depression between the trapezius muscles.

Ren 24 (Ghost Market)   In the depression in the center of the mentolabial groove.

PC 8 (Ghost Cave) On the transverse crease of the palm, between the second and third metacarpals. When the fist is clenched, the point is just below the tip of the middle finger.

Du 23 (Ghost Hall) 1 cun directly above the midpoint of the anterior hairline.

Ren 1 (Ghost Hidden)   Between the anus and the root of the scrotum in males or the posterior labial commisure in females.

LI 11 (Ghost Minister)   When the elbow is flexed, in the depression at the lateral end of the transverse cubital crease, midway between the biceps brachii tendon and the lateral epicondyle of the humerus.

Hai Qian (Ghost Seal) Between the frenulum and the tip of the tongue.

MYUNG KIM'S ACUPUNCTURE POINTS

1.   Yin/Yang paired channels of the arm. These are Qi supplying points for acute disease conditions of the three Yin organs.

Lung   LI 16

Heart   SI 11

Pericardium TW 15

2.   Connecting points of the Brother channels. These are used for external injuries.

Hand Yang Ming/Large Intestine Channel St 12

Foot Yang Ming/Stomach Channel   LI 15

Hand Tai Yang/Small Intestine Channel   UB 11

Foot Tai Yang/Urinary Bladder Channel   SI 15

Hand Shao Yang/Triple Warmer Channel   GB 21

Foot Shao Yang/Gall Bladder Channel   TW 15

3.   Back Shu (associated) and Front Mu (alarm) points of the Reproductive Organs

	BACK SHU	FRONT MU
Ovaries (Testes)	GB 30	Liv 12
Uterus (Prostate)	Reproduction Point *	Liv 11

* Locating the Reproduction Point-First, draw a horizontal line from GB 30 to the Du (GV) Channel. Then, follow the outside UB Channel down to a point slightly below UB 54. The intersection of these two lines is the Reproduction Point.

The following three points are only used when there is a blockage of Qi in their Channel. They are especially useful when one side is more obstructed than the other.

4. Small Intestine Channel Extra Point

Located between SI 8 and SI 9, halfway between the elbow and the axillary fold beside the medial aspect of the humerus bone. It is closer to the armpit than Heart 2. The exact location varies from person to person. In the case of a person with neck pain, the pain will radiate down from the GV (Du) Channel to UB 11 and across to SI 15. From there the pain can radiate down the SI Channel from SI 14 to SI 1.

5. Kidney Channel Extra Point

Located between Kidney 10 and Kidney 11. It is posterior to Liver 10 and 11 and close to the anus. It will appear when there are Kidney organ or channel problems or when there is severe Liver Qi Stagnation that manifests at Liver 10 and 11.

6. Spleen Channel Extra Point

Located between Spleen 11 and Spleen 12 and near either Liver 10 or Liver 11. It will appear when there are Spleen organ or channel problems or when there is severe Liver Qi Stagnation that manifests at Liver 10 and 11.

PROPORTIONAL MEASUREMENTS

Cun : A unit of measurement used to locate points. The length of one cun depends upon the body shape of the individual patient as well as the part of the body being measured.

The distance from the anterior to the posterior hairline is 12 cun. When measuring someone who has a receding hairline or is bald, use the distance between the glabella (between the eyebrows) and the external occipital protuberance. This is 14 cun.

The distance between the nipples is 8 cun.

From the navel to the upper border of the symphisis pubis is 5 cun.

Between the sterno-costal angle and the navel is 8 cun.

The distance between the medial border of the scapula and the center of the spine is 3 cun.

From the end of the axillary fold at the armpit to the transverse cubital crease at the elbow is 9 cun.

From the transverse cubital crease to the transverse carpal crease at the wrist is 12 cun.

Between the level of the upper border of the symphisis pubis and the medial epicondyle of the femus along the inner thigh is 18 cun.

Between the prominence of the great trochanter and the level of the middle of the patella (kneecap) along the outer thigh is 19 cun.

From the level of the middle of the patella to the tip of the lateral malleolus (ankle bone) is 16 cun.

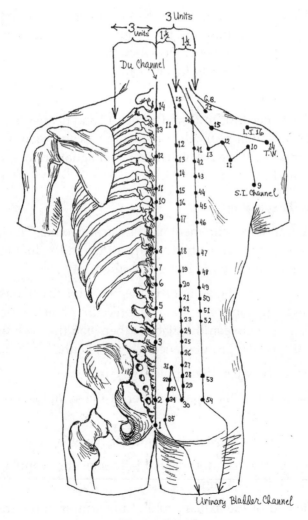

Figure 10-33

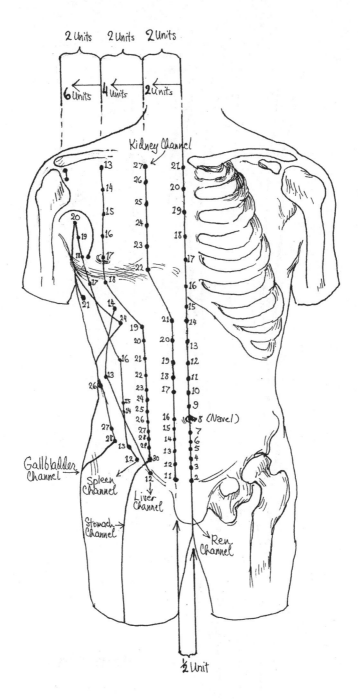

Figure 10-34

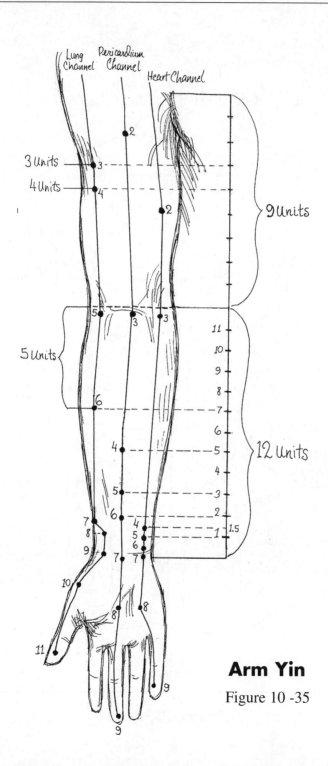

Arm Yin

Figure 10 -35

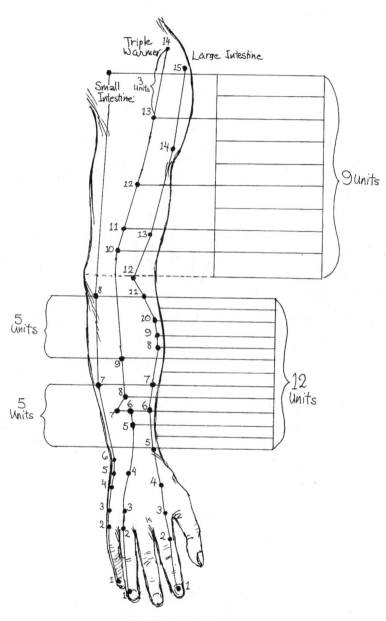

Arm Yang

Figure 10 -36

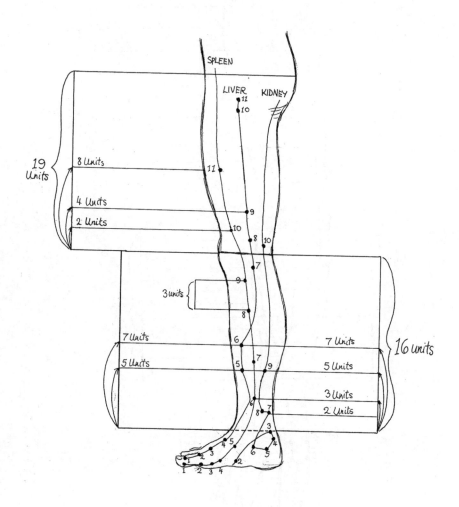

Leg Yin

Figure 10 -37

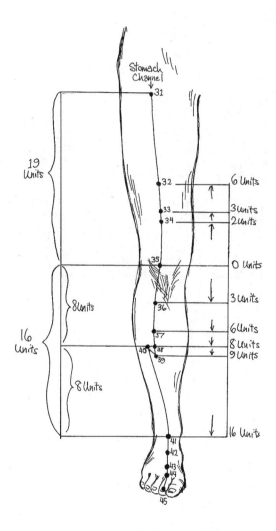

Stomach

Figure 10 -38

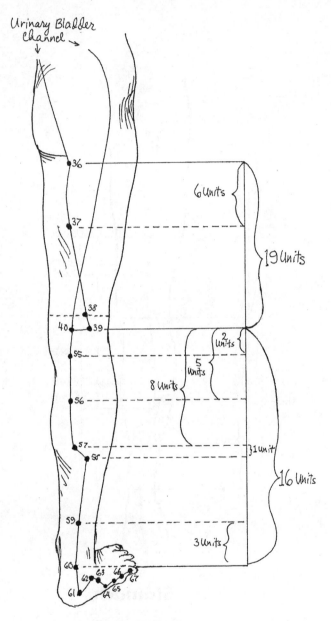

Leg Urinary Bladder

Figure 10 -39

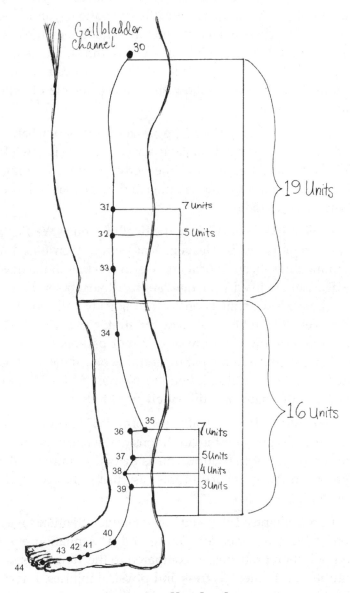

Leg Gall Blader

Figure 10 -40

Yin/Yang Theory and My Method of Acupuncture Treatment

"What style of acupuncture do you practice?" I have been asked this question by many acupuncturists, patients, and even by students and teachers at an acupuncture school here in New England. Some people have labelled my style as Taoist, others as a Martial Arts style, but I do not really follow any one particular style of acupuncture. I merely follow the main principle of acupuncture-Yin/Yang Theory.

In 169 AD, Zhang Zhong Jing was the major of Changsha, a city in the northern part of China. He wrote Shang Han Lun (Treatise on Cold-Induced Diseases) and the herbal formulas outlined in this book were used throughout China and indeed are still used to treat many diseases today.

Almost 1000 years later, in the twelfth century, Ye Tien Si (whose Taoist name is Leave, Heaven, Man) wrote Wen Bing Lun, which examined the effects of heat and warm weather in the development of disease. He lived near the Yangtze River in southern China. In this climate, severe infections spread quickly and could prove toxic. They were difficult to treat using the strategies of Zhang Zhong Jing. Ye observed how exposure to different pathogens caused specific epidemic diseases, anticipating germ theory in the West. He formulated new herbal prescriptions to counter febrile diseases, which like those of Zhang are still widely used today.

Why did Ye Tien Si create new formulas? He figured out that the formulas designed for the conditions of the north did not directly fit the conditions of the south. This is a good example of the application of Yin/Yang Theory, in this case using the North/South relationship.

In this chapter I devoted considerable attention to an explanation of the Yin (Oriental) culture and its sanitation, malnutrition, and pollution problems, as compared to the Yang (Western) culture with its severe mental stress and physical injuries. I have also discussed how my acupuncture style is based in the traditions of the East as modified to the conditions of the West-again simply an application of Yin/Yang Theory.

Japanese acupuncture emphasizes palpation of the stomach area (Yin part of the body) as a means of diagnosis and treatment and does not focus on the back (Yang part) of the body. When treating women's gynecological problems with the Chinese style an acupuncturist usually treats points on the Spleen Channel. But as I have emphasized in this chapter, problems in the Gall Bladder and Liver Channels are more prevalent in the US and these channels should be treated if American women encounter gynecological problems.

Vice President Al Gore visited China in the first part of 1997. He found that about 75% of the drinking water was contaminated and that severe air pollution due to all the homes burning coal for heat in the winter and cooking year round was causing a high incidence of lung disease. I am sure he saw the sanitation and malnutrition problems which cause Lung and Spleen problems (digestion and absorption problems and gynecological problems caused by Blood Deficiency.) In short, he saw that contemporary Chinese health problems involve the hand Tai Yin Lung Channel and the foot Tai Yin Spleen Channel. That is why to this day Chinese acupuncturists teach treatment for these channels, no matter what country they practice in.

Why have most acupuncturists failed to adapt their skills to their environment? The answer is simple. They learned their method from Chinese, Korean, or Japanese teachers or masters who teach "this is the truth, this is the way." Also many acupuncturists have been trained in mathematics, computer science, physics, and chemistry, "exact sciences" which are not open to interpretation. What they do not realize is that Yin/Yang Theory can and should be applied to acupuncture treatment anywhere in the world.

One example of this is the fire acupuncture technique, which was passed down by my ancestors over thousands of years to me. When I practice fire acupuncture on the back of a patient, after I insert the needle I apply fire in the form of a cigarette lighter. I discovered that this technique can be adapted for the season, location, and for each individual.

Fire technique can be applied to patients living in the northern portion of the United States and in Canada, where the climate is very cold and windy during the winter months, comparable to Mongolia and North Korea, where the technique was developed. I could also apply this technique in Antarctica and southern South America, as well as anywhere at high altitude. It is also appropriate where air conditioning is extensively used. I used the fire technique more in the winter than the summer, and more with older than younger patients.

Understanding this application is not really difficult. We see it every day of our lives, for example with what we buy. Cars made by Volvo are very popular in the northern and Rocky Mountain regions of the United States which have climates similar to Sweden, where Volvos are made. People in Florida and California do not buy this type of car, opting for American-made convertibles, which are more suited to their climate.

The existentialist philosophers Albert Camus (1013-1960) and Jean-Paul Sartre (1905-1980) believed that the source of worry for man was that because he was totally free and responsible for his actions he felt overwhelmed by new situations and choices. They should have learned and applied the theory of Oriental Medicine: Yin/Yang and adaptability.

Chapter 11

Cancer & Oriental Medicine

W estern medicine believes that pollutants, intake of carcino-gens, and inherited genes cause cancer. According to Oriental Medicine, cancer is caused by factors that cause Qi stagnation, including weather, emotions, injury, and nutrition (see Chapter 4). Cancer patients in mainland China, India and the Third World countries of Asia believe their cancer problems are mainly due to malnutrition, sanitation, and pollution.

As I mentioned in the introduction, Asian cultures (Yin cultures) are based on agricultural societies, which are relatively less mobile than the West. In contrast, American culture (a Yang culture) is rel-atively more nomadic. In the U.S., 50 million people move every year, causing significant socioeconomic problems and emotional stress. For children, this means adaptation to a new home, school, friends, and possibly a new climate. Home town community val-ues, familiar doctors, pastors, and teachers no longer exist.

The physical act of moving causes spinal strain and injuries. In the U.S., car accidents account for 2 million injuries and 40 thousand deaths each year. Seventy million other injuries occur each year in the U.S., and 20 million of these injuries cause disabilities. In addi-tion, 50 million surgeries are performed each year. Thus, each year 20% of the U.S. population moves and 20% undergo surgery, while 20% of the population suffers chronic back pain.

Excluding a few industrialized countries, the life style in most Asian countries has changed little in the past 100 years. Americans, in contrast, live with more stress than any other country; this is due to stress from work, family dysfunction, and injuries caused by machines and tools, automobile accidents, and gunshots.

I remember that when I first came to the U.S. in 1970 I was sur-prised to see how American children built their snowmen. As you know, an American snowman usually has three parts: a large base, a smaller trunk, and a still smaller head. In Asia, we built snowmen in two parts: a head and a body.

Another new thing I encountered here was chiropractors. I had never seen one in Korea. Today this has changed. There are some chiropractors in South Korea, and more Koreans are coming to the United States to study this profession. I believe that chiropractic medicine was more widely practiced here than in Korea simply because most Caucasian Americans are much taller than the average Asian. This additional height leads to more strain on the neck and lower back, as well as more susceptibility to injury in those areas. In addition, Caucasian Americans are more prone to osteoporosis as they age than are Asians because of the additional stress on their bones. In light of these facts, it is interesting that the American snowman is divided both at the neck and the lower trunk/back, while the Asian snowman is not.

As the economies of East Asia develop, the average size of the people increases. After years of war, malnutrition, poor sanitation and widespread health problems, the average Korean in the 1950s stood about 5' 5," or 165 cm. Since the new generation of Koreans who have grown up since 1970 are far better fed than their parents, Koreans are now almost as tall as Caucasian Americans. As a result, there are many more neck and back injuries due to sports, car accidents, and other causes. Thus, my diagnostic method will become increasingly popular in South Korea as I emphasize examining parts of the body that are stressed by this new growth spurt. Of course, these growth-related problems do not exist in North Korea; people there are still shorter and have fewer spinal injury problems than in the South. In the North, the main problem is malnutrition.

Some observers of modern China have suggested that as the country becomes more industrialized it will decrease the area devoted to agriculture while its population continues to increase. If true, China would have to increase its imports of grain from the U.S. This would affect other grain-importing countries like Korea and Japan. Since prices would increase to reflect increased demand, Korea would not be able to import as much grain as it needed. Thus, by the next century people in Korea would again be shorter; visits to the chiropractor and my diagnostic method would then lose popularity. As Yin/Yang theory states, everything continues to change according to time and place.

Americans are watching increasingly violent movies. Since they are bored with the one-to-one duels of cowboy Western movies, the spaghetti Westerns have been replaced by movies showing massive violence. Detective movies and video games showing violent Oriental martial arts scenes are popular, and some violent videos are shown on virtual reality devices. People enjoy watching boxing, wrestling matches, and car racing with accidents — ways to relieve their stresses by using their sadistic nature. These types of excited and violent emotions, like injury scars, will block the Qi circulation in the human body.

Cancer is caused by emotional characteristics and body type as well as carcinogens (from air, food, and water pollution) and genetic inheritance. Body type problems include increased injuries to the neck and lower back in very thin people, and tall people are prone to spinal injury. People can inherit emotional sensitivity, which may result in stomach ulcers, ulcerative colitis, stomach cancer and other digestion-related problems (see previous chapters for discussions of other organs and emotional relationships).

Organs that have genetic flaws can also cause cancer and other diseases. Sometimes I have encountered mothers and daughters with similar problems: body pain on the same side, the same kind of emotional sensitivity and related problems. They would both have neck pain that radiated to the left shoulder and the left side of the small finger of the small intestine channel. Gall bladder channel problems also show up on the same side in both patients.

My experience with many patients leads me to believe that surgery scars will block Qi flow on the side of the body with the scar and could result in tumor growth. An appendectomy scar (on the right side) will affect the right breast, right ovary, and right testicle functions. My theory is that the Qi flow can be stimulated with acupuncture and thereby prevent the tumor.

I consider surgery scars and physical injuries, especially spinal injuries that cause Qi stagnation to acupuncture channels, to have the same effect as attacking acupuncture points or pressure points with fingers to paralyze opponents in martial arts. These martial arts blows will not only bring pain and paralysis to the attacked area, they will also cause Qi stagnation to the designated acupuncture channel, leading to permanent injury or even death. In 1971 I published a book, "Acupuncture for Self Defense," which described in detail the attack and treatment methods. I recommended that most injured persons should be treated by acupuncture. This book is out of print now, but I will revise it soon.

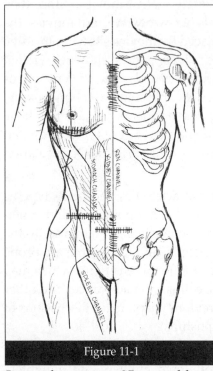

Figure 11-1

I would like to describe two case histories to illustrate how surgical scars can lead to tumors. A 27 year-old patient had an appendectomy scar when he was 14 years-old and his right testicle became smaller than his left testicle. Ten years later a doctor found a tumor in his right testicle. In another case, a 35 year-old woman with an ovarian tumor on her right side had undergone an appendectomy five years ago. The appendectomy scar had blocked Qi flow in the area and the acupuncture channels around it. A few years later intestinal adhesion and pain recurred. I treated her successfully with acupuncture, and her pain has disappeared.

Cesarean section procedures can also block the flow of Qi. I do not want to argue about the necessity of Cesarean section in this country. In 1996, 25 percent of all babies will be born in the U.S. through C-section. The occurrence of the procedure seems to increase each year. As shown in diagram 11-1, the surgeon makes a small incision, about one inch (2.5 cm) just above the pubic hair and around acupuncture points REN 2 and 3. The doctor then makes an invisible incision about 5-6 inches (12-15 cm) horizontally in about 90 percent of the cases. If fat and thick muscles develop around the uterus, the surgeon will make a 5-6 inch (12-15 cm) incision vertically. After the baby is born, the scar will shrink gradually to half its size or less. The scar will affect Qi flow in the Ren channel. As a result, abdominal pain, digestive problems and menstrual problems can occur (see figure 11-1).

I would like to cite some additional case studies to illustrate my point. Nancy O. was a 48 year-old woman who had delivered three babies through three vertical cesarean sections at ages 24, 31, and 38. Seven years later she developed pericarditis. A hole in the wall of her heart was discovered, which was corrected with surgery. However, she got tired very easily. I treated her heart and Ren channels with acupuncture and herbs. Her condition improved after a few treatments.

In another case, Ellen M., a 37 year-old woman, had a thyroid problem that caused an egg-sized swelling in the right side of her neck. This swelling blocked her swallowing ability, resulting in a build-up of saliva that needed to be removed with a syringe. After a second episode, her physician recommended removal of the thyroid gland.

When she came to me for treatment, I discovered that she had delivered two babies through vertical cesarean section and had a cesarean section abortion. She suffered from right side gall bladder channel problems. This affected the right side of her body, including the right side of her neck. After I performed a few treatments of acupuncture, her swollen thyroid gland disappeared.

I would like to cite a case of a male patient with Qi obstruction due to surgery. John D., a 28 year-old male, complained of pain in his left eye. Upon examination I discovered injuries from a motorcycle accident that happened two years ago. Because of right shoulder muscle damage, tissue had been surgically removed from his left leg around the GB 31 point area and transplanted to the damaged shoulder muscle. His left testicle was underdeveloped, and he complained of pain in this area as well. The surgery caused gall bladder channel blockage. The effects of damage to this channel are not well known to Western medical practitioners.

LIVER & GALLBLADDER CHANNEL PROBLEMS

It is my belief that liver and gall bladder channel problems are the major problems facing people in the twentieth century. Since they tend to suffer more mental stress than in previous eras, modern people are more susceptible to liver Qi stagnation than their ancestors. Mental stress can also impede recovery from disease. For example, if two healthy patients of the same age both suffer from Hepatitis C infection, the patient with less mental stress is more likely to be cured than the other.

"Liver Qi stagnation"[38] not only depresses the functioning of the liver, but also disturbs Qi flow in the liver, gall bladder, triple warmer and pericardium channels. It will especially affect the gall bladder channel and cause: stiffness in the knee (GB 31, 32, 33), waist, thigh and hip area (GB 30); breast pain during PMS or during menses (GB 21, 22); stiffness in the shoulder and neck (GB 21); stiffness between the backside of the ear and the base of the skull beside the trapezius muscle (GB 20, GB 12); blurry eyes, painful eyes (GB 1); and temporal headache (GB 2, 3). If a patient with the above condition is then injured on the lumbar spine or on the ankle, this injury will add "insult to injury." If there is a vertebral disk compress on either the right or left side of the nerve along the spine, the patient will feel more pain on one side than on the other side. Few patients would feel pain alternately on the right or left side.

If a patient complains of left eye pain, double vision, and/or watery eye, he or she may have problems in the left knee, hip and ankle. The left GB 37 (Kwang Ming-brighter eye) will have more pain than the identical point on the other side of the leg. This type of patient would be more susceptible to frostbite on the 4th toe and the 4th finger when exposed to the cold. If this condition goes untreated for a long time, it will become a chronic problem. Then the patient will experience cold legs, cramps and atrophy in one leg, which will become smaller than the other and will have more cramps, cold and pain. If exposed to air conditioning or cold wind in the summer time, the patient should cover himself or herself with a blanket.

If one complains about blurry eye or eye pain in both eyes, these would be considered to be caused by liver Qi stagnation. Liver Yang rising affects both sides evenly. If one is injured on the gall bladder channel and does not show any problem at one side of the eye, it means that the problem is very mild or that the injury happened not long ago.

If a patient has a sinus infection (sinusitis), it will disturb the Qi flow to one side of the eye when there is pre-existing Qi stagnation of the stomach, gall bladder, urinary bladder or the liver channels. If a patient has pain at GB 30 on the hip, one will also feel pain on the opposite side (Liver 12) on the groove. This will affect ovary function and cause infertility. If pain occurs all the time, not only at menstruation, I suspect the woman probably has an ovarian tumor. If she has pain at GB 31, 32, and 33, she will also have pain at Liver 9, 10, 11. This will disturb the uterine function and can cause endometriosis, vaginitis, uterine tumors, miscarriage and other gynecological problems. In Western gynecology physicians normally use their fingertips to feel ovarian tumors. However, I recommend my method for every female patient. First use finger pressure on GB 30, 31, 32, and 33 and Liver 9, 10, 11, and 12. Second, ask whether pain occurs during menstruation or all the time, especially on GB 30 and Liver 12. If pain exists on GB 30 and Liver 12 all the time, then an ovarian tumor will be suspected. The patient should then see a gynecologist for a laproscopy exam.

Sometimes ultrasound exams can detect only tumors in the uterus, but not ovarian tumors. Even if a tumor is not found in the ovary, there will be hormonal imbalance, infertility and susceptibility to tumors in the future.

If a patient has a gall bladder channel problem at GB 30 and lower back pain on one side, it will affect the dai[39] channel (belt) of GB 26, 27 and 28 of the same side. If the condition gets worse, the patient will develop organ prolapse and hernia on the same side. If there is severe pain, especially at GB 28, there is an increased likelihood of prolapse of the uterus.

If one considers the ear as a center point, then the gall bladder and triple warmer channels circulate around the head four times and eight times, respectively, on both sides of the head. Qi is supplied to the pituitary gland, the pineal gland and the hypothalamus. If Qi flow is disturbed, then the patient will lose control of hormonal production, body temperature, appetite, and sensitivity to light. If the patient has been suffering severe mental stress and injury along the pericardium, triple warmer, gall bladder and liver channels for a long time, the patient may be particularly susceptible to brain tumors.

Any Qi flow blockage at GB 21 points (between the shoulder and neck) will affect TW 15 (just above the scapula) and will go down through the triple warmer channel. From GB 1 (just beside the lateral end of the eye) to TW 23 (just beside the lateral end of the eyebrow) the disturbance in Qi flow can cause pain at TW 17 (behind the ear lobe). Sometimes the result will be ear pain, ear infections, hearing difficulty, deafness, Meniere's disease, and vertigo. A patient with pain at GB 30, Liver 12 and/or GB 31, 32, Liver 9, 10 and 11 will be more vulnerable at one side of the ankle or knee. In addition, he or she may be more susceptible to testicular tumor, undersized testicles, or breast, eye, ear, or brain tumors. In the case of a diminished testicle, if one squeezes both testes, the patient will feel pain on the underdeveloped side. If the pain is severe, one can be susceptible to a tumor on that side.

I would like to offer a few additional examples from my practice to show how diseases can be addressed by diagnosing and treating gall bladder channel problems. First, I cite Mrs. S.Y. Han, a 25 year-old Asian college student who complained of a sprain in her right ankle. I asked her: "Do you have lower back pain?" "Why do you ask?" she replied. I said: "I believe a normal adult does not injure her ankle easily."

In Oriental Medicine, any knee or lower extremity injury could be caused by a lower back problem. Upon examination, I found that she had gall bladder channel problems. I explained that it could cause illnesses such as ovarian and breast tumors, eye problems, or vertigo. I also said that if a patient has a constant and severe headache, it may indicate a brain tumor. She cried and told me that on one side she had ovary and breast tumors removed and that she still had a brain tumor. She complained of vertigo and stated that sometimes she falls. I have been treating her, and her conditions are improving.

I have found that by palpating points on the liver and gall bladder channels, many problems in the body can be identified including breast, ovary, uterine, testicular and prostate tumors and cancers. I have yet to discover the points which can be used to indicate developing brain tumors which are often asymptomatic by the methods of Western Medicine until they are far advanced.

I have known patients with severe chronic headaches over many years who also had liver and gall bladder channel problems, yet an MRI test was always negative and no tumors were ever found. Conversely, some women I have seen had no headaches but did exhibit multiple liver and gall bladder channel problems with brain tumors. So the relationships are not yet clear between the liver and the gall bladder channels and brain tumors. I am confident that points will eventually be identified which can better predict a patient's prognosis.

But for now, all I can predict is that severe gall bladder channel problems on the right side can occasionally cause brain tumors on the right side. The same holds true for the left side.

In another case, Mrs. M. F. Young, an Asian woman married to a French man, complained of vertigo and Meniere's disease. The mother of a two year-old and six year-old, she fell down about once a month for the past ten years. She could not find any doctors in France to properly treat her. Upon examination, her lower back pain was found to radiate down to her leg through the gall bladder channel. This gall bladder channel problem caused twitching and, on occasion, double vision in her eye. (Gall bladder channel problems affect the triple warmer channel, which affects the balancing apparatus in the ear. The result is vertigo and Meniere's disease.) I have been treating her for the past two years with success; her double vision has disappeared and she has not fallen down again.

John D. also complained of eye problems, including double vision and a headache in the left temporal area. His left eye was smaller than his right eye, and his sinus infection only affected his left eye. In addition, his left eye sometimes twitched. I discovered he had a left shoulder injury about ten years ago and currently has a lower back problem with Qi stagnation in the gall bladder channel. The GB 37 point on his left leg, the Kwang Ming-brighter eye point found just above and outside the ankle bone, was more sore on his left side than on his right. I treated him ten times, and his condition improved greatly.

Marie S., another case from my practice, was a 40 year-old female who complained of severe shoulder and ear pain on her left side. Upon examination, she showed gall bladder channel problems on her left side. A surgeon had removed a cancer-like tumor from her left breast and ovary four years ago. I treated her regularly for six months, and I believe she is now free of any problems.

Another patient, Cecile R., complained of severe migraine headaches for the past twelve years. She had an ear canal problem when she was seven and has had lower back pain. I discovered that she has gall bladder channel problems. Unfortunately, a Western physician had injected cortisone in both of her GB 30 points (on her hips) twice. I recommended that she have many acupuncture treatments. I regret that this patient moved away before she had sufficient treatment. She will probably develop a brain tumor and ovarian cancer in the near future. Her case was a very interesting one. The injection of cortisone into her acupuncture point probably blocked Qi flow more severely than in any other case during my professional career.

In mainland China, doctors sometimes inject antibiotics on the acupuncture channel, claiming that this method can cure infections with a very low dosage. More research is needed to determine whether this method affects the acupuncture channel and whether the channel and the antibiotics work together.

Carol S., a 44 year-old mother of four children, presented another interesting case of gall bladder channel disorder. She complained of right ovary pain and had a hernia just below the naval near her pubic hair. As a result of ectopic surgery while pregnant in 1978, she had a four-inch long horizontal scar just below the umbilicus. Upon examination, I discovered she had a gall bladder channel problem on her right side that had existed for many years. During one winter she had eaten a diet consisting only of cold salad and did some heavy lifting. The lifting caused a midsection intestinal hernia. Her GB 26, 27, and 28 points (the dai-belt channel) were very tender. This weakness can result in hernia and a tilted uterus. The patient told me that doctors of Western medicine had diagnosed her tilted uterus. I treated her with acupuncture and herbal medicine about ten times. She is now free from ovarian pain.

In another case, a 54 year-old woman named Sandra complained of gall stone pain that began two months earlier and digestive problems that troubled her for the past 10 years. The Western medical diagnosis for her problems was cholecystitis, and she needed a cholecystectomy (excision of the gall bladder). She came to me because she was afraid of surgery and wanted to keep her organ. She had lower back pain, which radiated to the right side of the gall bladder channel.

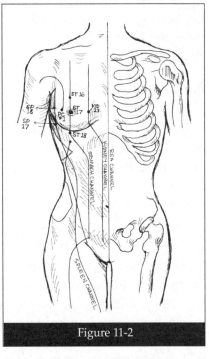

Figure 11-2

Jean, a 33 year-old woman, had similar problems. She had been previously diagnosed with Ewing's sarcoma (an endothelial myeloma that forms a fusiform swelling on a long bone. In her case it was her tibia). She underwent surgery, and a few months later she had chemotherapy and radiation therapy. Jean had a long history of lower back pain and gall bladder channel problems.

Valerie, a 30 year-old woman, also had cancer problems related to the gall bladder channel. Her ovarian and uterine cancer was surgically removed, followed by chemotherapy and radiation therapy. My examination revealed both lower back pain and gall bladder channel problems. Her health had worsened because she jogged regularly, even in cold wind and rain, blocking the Qi flow in her liver channel. Her mother, incidentally, had similar health problems, including ovarian and uterine tumors that had been surgically removed.

Gall bladder channel problems can cause cancer in the reproductive areas of men as well as women. For example, Mr. Johnson visited my clinic and complained about problems encountered after prostate cancer surgery. The cancer had been diagnosed by Western medicine three years earlier. He worried about the recurrence of cancer following prostate surgery. Twenty years ago he had undergone surgery, and ten years later he had inguinal hernia surgery. My examination detected gall bladder and liver channel problems. In addition, I found the hernia surgery had caused Qi stagnation in his Ren channel, which is directly related to the prostate gland. I have been treating him with acupuncture, herbs, moxa treatments, and Qi Gong exercises. I believe his prognosis is very good.

BREAST CANCER IN WOMEN

Any channel blockage resulting from a back injury or a surgical scar (after an appendectomy, Cesarean section, or other operations) can cause breast cancer. An appendectomy would tend to cause an ovarian or breast tumor on the right side. (Keep in mind that although this section refers only to women, breast cancel can occur in men as well).

The breast area has many acupuncture points and channel passages; ST 16, ST 17, KID 23, PC 1, SP 17, SP 18 GB 22 and GB 23. These are the places where tumor and cancer cells grow. If a woman has breast reduction surgery or silicon implant breast surgery, the Qi flow of most of these six channels will be blocked. Many problems may follow, including breast cancer. If a patient has a pre-existing gall bladder channel problem on one side, the breast on that side will heal much slower than on the other side. If a patient has an appendectomy scar, the right side of the breast will heal more slowly than the left side. In the worst possible scenario, where the patient has an appendectomy scar and a gall bladder channel pain on the right side, cancer of the right breast may result.

Two of my cases illustrate how breast cancer can be caused by channel blockage problems. Bobby, a 51 year-old woman, had been treated for breast cancer by removal of her entire right breast, followed by chemo- and radiation therapy. She had a long history of lower back pain that radiated down to the gall bladder channel on her right side. Susan, a 56 year-old woman, had her ovarian cyst removed about twenty years ago and her right breast was also removed. This year, a CAT scan showed a tiny nodule on her right side lung. Upon examination, I found an injection scar from chemotherapy on the #2 point of her right lung channel. Both Bobby and Susan, and many other women, have developed cancer or tumors in the same location in the breast (see Figure 11-2). I have discovered that about 90 percent of women with breast cancer had gall bladder channel problems.

SELF DIAGNOSTIC METHOD FOR CANCER DETECTION

I would like to introduce you to a procedure that you can practice at home to determine whether you suffer from gall bladder and liver channel problems. First, lie down on your back (see Figure 11-3). In this position you can check GB 31 by pressing with the tip of your middle finger while you hold your arms in the "attention" position. Next, press underneath the outside ankle bone to check GB 40. Liver 8, 9, 10, and 11, all found on the inside of the thigh, should next be checked. Kidney 1 is found on the bottom of the foot, while kidney 3 is between the inside ankle bone and the Achilles tendon. You should also check bladder 60, located between the outside ankle bone and the Achilles tendon. While still lying on your back, you can also check Small Intestine 8 and Heart 3 at the elbow and Triple Warmer 4 at the wrist.

Next, bend your knees up so that the soles of your feet are flat on the floor (see Figure 11-4). This will relax your abdominal muscles, allowing you to check GB 28. This point is just above and inside your hipbone (anterior superior iliac spine), for possible hernia or tilted uterus problems. Also, check LIV 12 in the pubic region for potential ovary problems.

A number of points around the breasts can be palpated for potential tumor problems, including Spleen 18, Stomach 16-18, LIV 14, and GB 22-24. You should also check for sensitivity between the nipple and the REN meridian (on the midline of the body (see Figure 11-2). Male patients should squeeze both testes to check for any pain. Also, notice whether one testicle is smaller then the other one.

Next, you should turn over onto your stomach. In this position you can check GB 30, located on your hip (see Figure 11-5). If lying on your stomach causes discomfort, you can lie on your side and press one GB 30 at a time (see Figure 11-6). First, extend your smallest finger to the side and place it on the anus. Next, fold up the three middle fingers as if you were making a fist. Extend the thumb towards the hip (near the great trochanter bone). Then press down on the adjacent area and test for pain.

The prone position is the only way to check your lumbar area and neck for vertebral problems. Of course, this is fairly difficult to perform on yourself in any position. For more information on self-diagnosis, see Chapter 10, "Palpating Acupuncture Points for Diagnosis."

Problems are caused in the liver and gall bladder channels for several reasons. First, we have evolved during evolution from walking on four legs to walking upright. We then used our former forelegs as arms and created civilization with our two hands, as we learned in biology class. Our skeletal structure changed as part of this evolutionary process, but our upright carriage came at a cost — back problems. These problems of such ancient origin are often aggravated by pregnancy, and conditions are worsened when women are given lumbar area anesthesia during delivery. Furthermore, modern habits such as the wearing of high heeled shoes, especially while lifting heavy objects, can cause injuries in the second through fifth lumbar vertebrae.

Acupuncture doctors usually believe these problems start with sciatic pain running through the urinary bladder channel, then moving to the gall bladder channel; sometimes the pain originates in the gall bladder channel. Movement of problems through various channels is common with many contemporary illnesses, such as chronic fatigue syndrome and systemic lupus. The liver, gall bladder, triple warmer and pericardium channels are affected in these cases. Sometimes a problem in the urinary bladder channel affects the kidney, small intestine, and heart channels. In the worst cases, four, six, or all twelve channels are affected.

When discussing the causes and spread of channel-related illness, we need to mention the stress of modern life as a major factor. People are subjected to a higher level of stress now than at any previous time in history. This stress causes liver Qi stagnation, which then affects the gall bladder channel. Other distinctly modern factors cause problems, such as blood stagnation in the ovaries and uterus. These factors can be environmental (such as pollution or foodstuff contaminated by chemicals), hereditary (such as a gene that triggers cancer), or due to lifestyle choices. The intake of drugs, alcohol, or tobacco and sexual promiscuity are all lifestyle-related risk factors. Young women, who as a group are more likely than older women to have more than one sexual partner, are known to contract more venereal diseases (including herpes).

Adverse weather conditions, combined with modern fashion styles that don't adequately protect the body, can also cause problems. Exposure to cold rain, cold wind, and air-conditioned air can assault the groin area and cause Qi stagnation in the liver channel. The modern fashion of wearing shorts and short skirts even in cold weather can contribute to this problem. In Oriental Medicine this condition is called "cold stagnating liver channel."

I treated a young man for a cold weather-related problem caused by sports practice. Adbul K., a 16 year-old high school football player, complained about a stretching sensation and related pain in his penis and testes. I had given him two treatments for shoulder problems caused by football injuries. Upon examination, I could not find any lower back injuries or pulled muscles in his groin area. I then asked him if he practiced football in heavy rain, and he confirmed that his team practiced over the weekend in windy and cold rain. I treated him with hot needle acupuncture by heating the needle with fire. I also recommended that he use moxa treatment at home. After two acupuncture treatments, he was relieved of all pain.

Beside the conditions mentioned above, the pericardium, triple warmer, gall bladder, and liver channels can have problems as a result to chronic ankle or knee injuries. Also, any epidemic febrile disease can transmit heat through the above-mentioned channels and cause related problems.

Many gall bladder channel problems are preventable, including ailments caused by poor eating habits. Americans suffer from more of these problems than Asians do because they eat more fast food and dine at restaurants more frequently. Fried food causes many of these diet-related problems. Restaurants tend to re-use their frying oil, a particularly dangerous trend that leads to gall stone formation. Frequency of eating also affects the gall bladder channel. Americans contribute to their problems by failing to eat regularly three times a day, as their grandparents did when they were farming and hunting. Irregular eating does not provide the proper stimulation of the

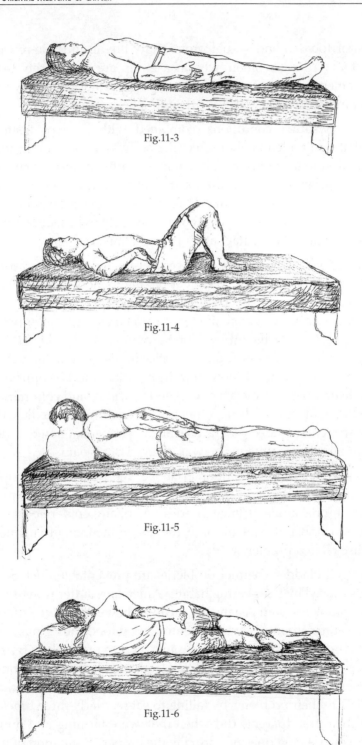

Fig.11-3

Fig.11-4

Fig.11-5

Fig.11-6

gall bladder.

About 500,000 gall bladder surgeries (cholecystectomies) are performed each year in the United States, providing one of the largest sources of hospital income today. I have developed a very good herbal tablet to treat some of these problems before they become acute, using an herbal formula handed down by my ancestors. The formula works much better when combined with acupuncture, but readers can use it along with the moxa self-treatments described in Chapter 9.

It is important to prevent and care for problems in the gall bladder channel or other channels because they are connected to one another. The gall bladder, triple warmer, pericardium and liver channels are located in the middle of the other channels (see Figures 10-11, 10-12, 10-13). Therefore, Qi stagnation in any of these channels will affect the channels that cross them horizontally, creating additional Qi stagnation and deficiency.

Here are a few examples of channel interdependency. Any Qi stagnation in the urinary bladder channel will affect the gall bladder channel, since Qi flowing in the outer branch of the urinary bladder channel passes through GB 30 on the cheeks of the hip (see Chapter 10, section on Qi passage). I have also observed that left side gall bladder channel problems easily affect several organs, including the heart, left lung, and kidney. Right side gall bladder channel problems easily affect the gall bladder, right lung, kidneys and liver organs (see Chapter 10, section on palpation diagnostic methods).

The 2,000 year-old book, *The Yellow Emperor's Internal Medicine*, states that all parallel acupuncture channels contain points that line up horizontally, perpendicular to the channels. If there is Qi stagnation in one point or in a Yang channel, it would affect the two nearest points in the two parallel Yang channels. The same rule applies to any Yin channels with Qi stagnation. For example, an injury at the 6th or 7th cervical vertebral area will cause a Qi disturbance at the urinary bladder point 1 around the eye through the urinary bladder channel. Alternatively, Qi stagnation could occur around the scapular area SI14 and SI15 up to the small finger through the small intestine channel. Qi stagnation might also go directly to the SI17 point under the angle of the mandible.

The examples cited above illustrate the Continuum of the Five Element Theory, which states that problems in one organ cause problems in the other organs. If Qi stagnation in an organ is not treated well or is never fully cured, it will result in a chronic problem and will develop into a disease involving many organs.

Cancer is an extremely serious problem in the United States and is far more prevalent that you might believe. Here are a few startling statistics: about 30 percent of women over 40 have some kind of tumor in their ovaries or uterus. About 50 percent of men and women over 50 have a polyp in their rectum. Furthermore, recent medical surveys discovered the following prevalence of prostate cancer: 20 percent of men in their 50's; 30 percent of men in their 60's; 40 percent of all men in their 70's; and 50 percent of all men in their 80's or older. Also, 7,200 men will get testicular cancer in the U.S. every year; 350 of them will die between the ages of 15 and 35. Although there are no statistics for concurrence of both polyp and prostate cancer, Oriental medical theory would predict they are likely to occur together. These diseases share common causes: Qi stagnation from lifestyle problems, emotional or physical injuries, or scars.

It has been predicted that during 1996, 14,000 people will die from ovarian cancer, 44,000 will die from breast cancer, 42,000 will die from prostate cancer, and 40,000 will die from lung cancer. There are no exact statistics on recurrence of cancer after surgery. The American Cancer Society estimates that 596,600 women in the United States will be diagnosed with cancer in 1997 and that 265,900 women will die from cancer this year; 764,300 men will be diagnosed and 292,300 men will die from cancer. Western medicine blames recurrence of cancer on the side effects of chemotherapy and radiation therapy. They do not consider that surgery scars, resulting in Qi stagnation in acupuncture channels, affect recurrence rates.

If you discover any symptoms after using the self-diagnostic methods in this book, you should see a Doctor of Oriental Medicine who specializes in both acupuncture and herbal medicine. At least, you should visit a licensed acupuncturist, apply moxa or warm water treatment, use herbal medicine, and practice Qi Gong breathing exercises.

Oriental Medicine, particularly herbs and acupuncture, should be used especially before and after surgery to help the patient recover more quickly. Many patients also find they get more emotional and physical support from a Doctor of Oriental Medicine, and have more energy from Oriental treatments than they do from Western medicine.

During chemotherapy and radiation therapy in China and Korea today, doctors commonly use small amounts of herbs. After chemotherapy, they use detoxification and Qi tonification herbs if a patient's cancer is not terminal or stomach cancer. In mainland China scientists have conducted much research on the subject of Oriental herbal medicine for treating cancer.

Although $30 billion has been spent for cancer research in the U.S. over the past 25 years, the cancer rate has not improved substantially. I believe it is time to look in other directions. It is time for "the wisdom of the Orient."

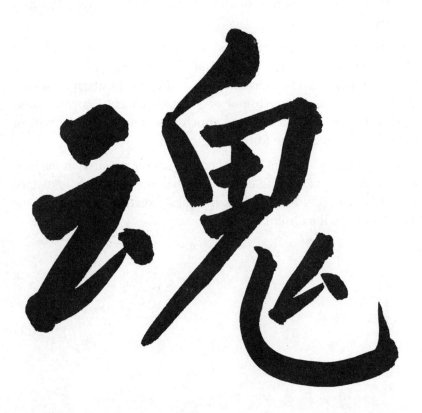

HUN

Chapter 12
Traditional Chinese Internal Medicine

In traditional Chinese medicine, internal organs are categorized as Yin or Yang. Solid organs are considered to be Yin and are called zang organs. These are the liver, heart, spleen, lung, kidney and pericardium. Hollow organs are considered Yang and are called fu organs. These are the gall bladder, small intestine, stomach, large intestine and urinary bladder.

In TCM theory, zang organs are the manufacturing organs. They store the jing, Qi, Blood and body fluid. The fu organs digest, absorb, transmit nutrients and excrete waste. TCM emphasizes the study of zang organ syndromes because most chronic diseases originate in zang organs. Acute diseases are usually started from the fu organs and are easier to treat than zang organ syndromes.

Oriental Medicine is based on understanding the nature of Qi , Blood, Yin and Yang and how they all relate to each other. These are the fundamentals of Oriental medical theory and it is essential to understand the different types of Qi, blood, Yin and Yang conditions in order to learn how to diagnose and treat a patient.

The treatments covered in this book involve acupuncture and moxibustion. As mentioned earlier, moxibustion is effective in curing chronic problems such as indigestion, coldness, numbness and weakness. Moxa is a tonification method which can be used by everyone. Acupuncture is most effective when treating acute problems such as severe pain or a heat condition such as fever but can also be used for acute or chronic conditions. Note that in the following section, reference will be made to the DU and the REN channels. The DU channel is also known as the Governing Vessel and the REN channel is also known as Conceptual Vessel.

Acupuncture point prescriptions in this chapter are based on TCM theory. The TCM theory concentrates principally on internal medicine and organ disorders. Over the past centuries, as well as today,

Oriental Medicine as practiced in Asian countries focused on treatment of internal organ diseases, including cancer, which were caused by poor sanitation, malnutrition and infection. Because of this, channel theory was de-emphasized in favor of a focus on organ pathologies. Five Element Theory, another important foundation of acupuncture as it is currently practiced both in Asia and the West, focuses primarily on the interactions between the organ systems. It also de-emphasizes the channel theory aspect of Oriental Medicine.

But as previously discussed, Western disease is more often caused by external forces, and contemporary American health problems cannot be treated according to strict TCM theory.

My Three Dimensional Four Inter-Channel Theory can be used to treat both internal organ pathologies and external injuries which cause channel blockages. A blockage in one channel, if not properly treated, can develop into a four-channel problem because of the Yin/Yang and sister/brother relationships between the channels as described in Chapter 10. Because of this, the Three Dimensional Four Inter-Channel Theory is the most complete system to use for diagnosis and prognosis. But, of course, other systems have their strong points and differing approaches to acupuncture may be combined. Practitioners are encouraged to employ aspects of this new method along with their current styles for maximum effectiveness of treatment.

There are no specific quantities or lengths of time mentioned for treatments. How long to use moxa or how many acupuncture treatments are needed, should they be combined and in what ratio are questions that will not be answered here. Treatment will vary with the patient and the severity of the condition. These answers will come with an experienced Doctor of Oriental Medicine. A layman can treat him or herself using indirect moxa in place of acupuncture.

After the first acupuncture treatment, most patients will feel good, however, some will feel tired or experience some pain afterwards if they were too tense or fatigued before the treatment. After an acupuncture treatment, a patient may become sick if he or she immediately stresses the body by arguing with someone, doing athletics or consuming alcohol. Older people or people with a weak Qi condition may experience a few days of fatigue after treatment.

These patients should receive moxa or Qi Qong Massage until their bodies become strong enough to receive acupuncture. The location of the acupuncture points can be found in Chapter 10.

QI SYNDROME

There are four types of Qi syndromes; Qi deficiency, Qi prolapse, Qi stasis and rebellious Qi.

1) QI DEFICIENCY SYNDROME

Qi deficiency will usually affect the patient's energy level. Typically, Qi deficiency means that the Qi does not reach the upper parts of the body to supply the internal organs. As a result, the Wei Qi does not close the pores to regulate the skin surface. This in turn may allow external influences to penetrate the body.

CAUSE

Qi deficiency may occur from old age, a chronic illness, irregular diet or malnutrition.

SYMPTOMS

Dizziness and vertigo

Listlessness and asthenia

Spontaneous sweating aggravated by physical activity

Shortness of breath

Indolence (speaks in a low voice if at all)

Tongue will be pale

Pulse will be weak

Shortness of breath may also occur because the general Qi or lung Qi is weakened.

TREATMENT

The treatment principle is to tonify and replenish the Qi. Treatment includes applying acupuncture or moxa to points of the affected organ using the tonification method; ST 36, LU7 and K3. Use no more than four needles.

2) QI PROLAPSE SYNDROME

CAUSE

This is a type of Qi deficiency syndrome. A prolapse of an organ occurs when the Qi does not ascend to the upper body as a result of chronic Qi deficiency.

SYMPTOMS

Sensation of prolapse

Dizziness and vertigo

Listlessness and Asthenia

Gastrosis

Prolapse of the uterus

Prolapse of the anus

The tongue will be pale and the pulse will be weak and sinking.

TREATMENT

Treatment of Qi prolapse involves raising and tonifying the Qi. Use acupuncture and moxa on upper body points including Du 20. Also treat ST36 and K3. If the patient is very weak, he or she may faint during treatment.

3) QI STASIS SYNDROME

CAUSE

This syndrome causes obstruction in the flow of Qi to certain parts of the body. It can be caused by either emotional or physical imbalance including mental or nervous tension, improper diet, external pathogen or internal injury.

Cold wind can attack the surface of the body or invade the stomach directly.

SYMPTOMS

Pain

Distention - Qi does not move smoothly

Movable pain

Feel better after moving bowels or urination

The tongue will be bluish dark in color or white (but dull or not shinny)

Pulse will be sinking and tight

Excess heat or mild heat may also cause Qi stasis. Many people will experience stomach gas as a result of nervousness.

Treatment

Treatment involves acupuncture to LIV3, ST36, LI4 and H7. It is also important for the patient to remove the stress and emotional difficulties the patient is experiencing.

4) Rebellious Qi Syndrome

Cause

Rebellious Qi can be caused by an excess syndrome. There may be a pathogenic attack causing retention of phlegm and/or damp retention in the lung. Rebellious Qi syndrome occurs from the derangement of Qi where the Qi moves in the wrong direction. Often, this can result from prolonged anger.

Symptoms

Rebellious Qi will affect the lung, stomach and liver. If the lungs are affected and the lung Qi cannot descend, the patient will develop a cough.

Irregular or excessive food intake will cause pathogenic conditions in the stomach where the stomach Qi does not descend. Rebellious Qi in the stomach causes hiccups, nausea and vomiting.

Emotional stress can cause liver Qi to rise. If there is liver fire, then bleeding from the Vagina may follow. Vertigo, dizziness, headaches, fainting and vomiting blood are symptoms of rebellious Qi in the liver.

In each case, the tongue will be pale and dull (similar to stasis). The pulse will be floating and tight.

Treatment

The treatment principle is to cause the Qi to descend. The most effective way to treat this syndrome is to apply acupuncture to treat the lower part of the body, specifically, ST36, LU 7, ST 40, LIV3, and LIV2.

BLOOD SYNDROME

There are two types of blood syndromes; blood deficiency and blood stagnation.

1. BLOOD DEFICIENCY

CAUSE

Blood deficiency can be caused by a chronic loss of blood, sudden loss of blood, spleen or stomach deficiency, or upset emotions. All these conditions cause the blood to be overly consumed which in turn, causes the deficiency.

SYMPTOMS

Shallow or pale complexion

Dizziness and vertigo, blurred vision

Insomnia, palpitations

Numbness of extremities

Amenorrhea, delayed menstrual period

Pulse is thready and weak

TREATMENT

Treatment is to tonify and nourish the blood. This is accomplished through acupuncture and moxa on the points related to the liver and heart. These would be UB15, UB18, SP6, Liv3 and H7. Moxa can also be applied to SP1.

2. BLOOD STAGNATION

a) Blood Stagnation Caused by Blood Deficiency

SYMPTOMS

Pale face

Dizziness and vertigo

Insomnia and palpitations

Pain in a fixed area

The tongue will be pale with red or purplish dots

Pulse will be wiry

TREATMENT

This syndrome is treated by nourishing and activating the blood. Acupuncture points: H7, SP6, LIV3 and H5. Do not apply acupuncture to SP10 unless the syndrome is the excessive type.

B) BLOOD STAGNATION CAUSED BY QI DEFICIENCY

This occurs when the body does not have enough power (Qi) to move the blood.

SYMPTOMS

Feelings of listlessness and asthenia

He or she may feel indolent and experience spontaneous sweating

There may also be pain which will become more acute when the painful areas are touched

The tongue will be pale with bluish tinge and purplish dots

Pulse will be weak and sluggish

TREATMENT

To treat blood stagnation caused by Qi deficiency, you must tonify the Qi and activate the blood. To do so, apply acupuncture to ST36, LIV3, K3, LIV8, LI4, H5.

C) BLOOD STAGNATION CAUSED BY PATHOGENIC COLD

SYMPTOMS

Pain relieved by warmth

Cold extremities

Yang Qi circulation blocked by cold

Pale and dull tongue

Pulse will be deep, tight and slow

TREATMENT

You would treat this problem by warming up the channels and activating the blood; LI4, ST36, REN6, SP6 and UB11. Apply moxa more than acupuncture.

d) Blood Stagnation Caused by Blood Heat

Symptoms

Pain relieved by cold

Fever

Epidemic disease with high fever

Hemorrhage, delirium, constipation

Dark red tongue

Rapid and thready pulse

With this syndrome, the patient will lapse into a coma if the heat attacks the pericardium.

Treatment

The method for treating the problem is to remove the heat and activate the blood. To do this, use no moxa. Apply acupuncture to SP9 and SP8. If the condition is severe, apply acupuncture to K1 for resuscitation. This will help the blood to circulate to the lower part of the body.

Liver

The liver is the storehouse of the soul and the blood. The liver maintains the harmony of the Qi by regulating Qi flow and acts as the decision maker for the body. The health of the liver can be seen primarily through the eyes, nails and tendons. An unhealthy liver can cause anger, stress and irritability. The liver and the gall bladder are closely associated and as the health of the liver goes, so goes the health of the gall bladder.

The idea of stress was popularized by Hans Selye (1896 - 1985). Hans Selye was a Hungarian born Endocrinologist who after reading *The Yellow Emperor's Internal Medicine* (*Neijing*) which was translated into Latin, studied emotional problems and its effects on the human body. In 1938 while doing research and experiments with animals, he developed what is now popularly known as the "Stress Theory." His theories included causes and the effects of stress.

As mentioned earlier, the liver is the "decision maker" of the body. In modern society, there are often many decisions to make. For example, just trying to decide which of the 500 television channels to watch can induce a certain amount of stress.

Liver problems may be congenital but are often a result of job related stress. Hepatitis is a liver ailment. A husband and wife contract Hepatitis A, B and C. The wife develops antibodies and never developed the symptoms. The husband develops antibodies for A and B but not C. Not developing these antibodies may be the result of stress weakening the liver.

1) LIVER QI STAGNATION

CAUSE

Liver Qi stagnation can be caused by suppression of emotions. This will stop the free flow of Qi and cause a lack of initiative and motivation.

SYMPTOMS

There will typically be pains in both sides of the neck, armpits, ribs on both sides and the on either side of the head. Liver Qi stagnation effects the Shao Yang Channel, specifically, the Gall Bladder and Triple Warmer. Aside from pains in the rib cage, the patient will experience migraine headaches and pains in the lymphatic gland.

The patient may also have a tightness in the chest, feeling of choking or being unable to breath and the plum pit phenomenon in the throat. The patient may sigh a lot, experience dizziness and have a bitter taste in the mouth. He or she may be irritable, frustrated, experience mental depression and move from one project to another without finishing the first. A female patient may have irregular menstruation or have pre-menstrual syndrome (PMS).

The pulse will be wiry, particularly the liver pulse. The tongue will appear normal but have a bluish cast.

TREATMENT

In general, applying acupuncture to LIV14, UB18, ST36, LIV3 and LI4 will alleviate liver Qi stagnation.

2) PLUM PIT IN THROAT

To the patient, this will feel like there is a plum seed stuck in the throat which cannot get spit out. It is generally caused by severe stress or a thyroid gland condition.

TREATMENT

Acupuncture to REN22, H7, LIV14 and UB18 will help this symptom.

3) LIVER AND STOMACH DISHARMONY - LIVER QI ATTACKS THE STOMACH

This is also caused by stress. Vomiting and indigestion can be the result of the stomach Qi going upward. It is commonly known as acid indigestion or reflux.

TREATMENT

Treat ST36, REN12, UB21, ST25, LIV14 and UB18 with acupuncture.

4) LIVER AND SPLEEN DISHARMONY - LIVER QI ATTACKS THE SPLEEN

This is a result of severe mental stress causing diarrhea, abdominal pain and weakness.

TREATMENT

Treat ST40, SP6, LIV14, UB18, REN12, UB20, ST25 and LIV13 with acupuncture.

5) LIVER FIRE RISING

CAUSE

Liver Qi stagnation can cause liver fire rising. It can also be brought about by long-term stress or depression or from dramatic emotional changes such as a death in the family, divorce, etc. Overindulging in drinking and smoking can also cause liver fire rising.

SYMPTOMS

The symptoms when liver fire goes to the gall bladder channel are:

Splitting head aches and Migraines

Dizziness

Red face

Dry mouth and throat

Nose bleeds

Blood in urine

Deafness - as fire goes up, ringing or roaring sound in ears

Painful read swollen eye lids, conjunctivitis

Excessive anger

Temporary blindness lasting for a few days to a few weeks

Irritability

Impatience

Frustration

Bitter taste in mouth

Insomnia

Constipation

Dark scanty urine

Pain in the ribs

Muscle spasms and eye or leg twitches

The tongue is red with a yellow coating and the pulse will be wiry and rapid at about 5 or 6 beats per breath.

Western symptoms include hypertension, high blood pressure and migraine headaches, bleeding in the stomach, conjunctivitis, Meniere's disease, dizziness, loss of balance and ringing in the ear.

TREATMENT

The treatment principle is to clear the liver heat and cool down the fire.

Acupuncture should be applied to GB20, LIV2 and GB24 for headaches. H7, P6, SP6, UB18, UB19 and GB12 are the treatment points for insomnia. If the patient has high blood pressure, the acupuncture treatment should be applied to GB20, ST36, LI11, LIV3, ST17, ST36, P6, SP6, DU20, LIV2 and ST9. For vertigo, DU20, TW17 and UB10 are the points to concentrate on.

6) LIVER YANG RISING

CAUSE

Liver Yang rising is a long term deficiency of kidney or liver Yin. In this case, the liver Yin is injured, caused by deficiency of heart blood. Heart Qi stagnation and or heart fire is typically the cause of liver Yang rising.

SYMPTOMS

Headaches

Dizziness and blurred vision

Sudden blindness

Bitter taste

Periodic hot flashes on the face

Liver Yin deficiency

Blood shot eyes

Anger

Depression

Haste

Jumpy, impatience and restlessness

The pulse will be fast and wiry and the tongue will be red on both edges with a yellow coat.

TREATMENT

The treatment principle is to nurture and calm the liver Yin and subdue the heat syndrome. The acupuncture points for the ear ringing symptom are GB20, TW17, TW3, LIV2, K3 and UB23.

Acupuncture to ST40 will help to clear the sight and hearing problems caused by a phlegm build up. For symptoms of the ear (aural vertigo or dizziness in the ear), treat GB20, LIV3, TW17, ST19. P6 and K3 will help to nourish the Yin. For the sudden blindness, treat GB20, UB1, ST1, UB18, UB23, LI4, ST36 and GB37. To relieve heat in the head or eyes, treat UB62, UB63 and UB67.

7) LIVER YIN DEFICIENCY

CAUSE

The kidney and liver work in conjunction with each other. The kidney jing produces blood which in turn is used to nourish the liver; kidney Yin nourishes liver Yin. When this process is out of balance and the liver Yin does not receive enough nourishment and liver Yin deficiency is the result.

SYMPTOMS

False heat

Nighttime sweating

Restlessness

Insomnia

Dizziness

Muscle spasms, twitching

Ringing in the ears

Menopause

Dry red eyes (like to wear sunglasses)

The muscle spasms are a result of the tendons not receiving enough nourishment of Yin. The tongue will be red and thin and the pulse will be rapid and thready.

Western symptoms include infectious hepatitis, high blood pressure, hemiplegia or dry mouth and dizziness after a stroke which resulted in paralysis.

TREATMENT

Acupuncture should be applied to UB18, SP6, UB23, LIV2, LIV8, REN4, K3 and K7.

8) Liver Blood Deficiency

Cause

Liver blood deficiency can be caused by hemorrhage, trauma, or with women, profuse menstruation. Chronic illness may also cause spleen deficiency where nutrients are not absorbed.

Symptoms

The blood supply to the brain will be diminished causing dizziness. This same lack of blood to the head will cause blurred or hazy eye sight and black spots when the eyes are undernourished. Often, undernourished tendons will cause twitches and spasms. Since the liver is the store house of blood, liver blood deficiency may cause the menstrual cycle to be between 35 and 40 days, cause Amenorrhea or an irregular cycle, fear and timidity. The pulse will be superficial and hollow or slender and weak. The tongue will be pale as will the face and finger nails.

Treatment

Tonification and nurturing the blood is the key to treating this problem. To relieve the Amenorrhea, acupuncture should be applied to UB23 to tonify the kidney and REN 7. Also, apply acupuncture to SP6, UB17, SP10, ST30, SP8 to regulate menses and LIV8 to disperse Qi.

9) Liver Wind

There are two types of liver wind, internal and external. If the patient is suffering from external wind, the result is usually a tremor and spasm on the neck and back only. Internal wind is more serious and if left untreated can lead to paralysis. Phlegm is usually associated with liver wind. It will disturb the Qi flow causing tremors, convulsions, epilepsy, hemiplegia, Parkinson's disease and paralysis. Excessive consumption of alcohol and fatty food could create phlegm and heat in the body which can also trigger wind condition in liver.

Etiology

Liver fire rising

Liver Yang Rising - Uncontrollable Convulsions

External Heat Invade Internal - Injure Liver Yin

Yin Deficiency - Causes Tremors

Blood Deficiency - Causes Spasm

Qi Stagnation - Becomes Liver Fire and Triggers Liver Wind

SYMPTOMS

Uncontrolled tremors

Difficult speech

Stiff neck

Pulsating headache (comes and goes)

Extreme dizziness

Ringing in the ears

Facial rigidity

Paralysis

Profuse phlegm (when there is wind)

Unconsciousness and coma

Blurred vision

Opisthotonos

a) Wind With Liver Heat

If the patient has wind with liver heat, he or she will exhibit high fever, convulsions in the four limbs, contusions and clenched mouth, lips and hands, a red tongue and a rapid and wiry pulse.

b) Wind With Up Rising Liver Yang

If the patient has wind with up rising liver Yang, then there will be numbness, distortion of the mouth and eyes, dizziness and headaches. The tongue will be red and the pulse will be rapid and wiry.

c) Yin Deficiency with Wind

Where there is Yin deficiency with wind, the patient will have tremors (indicating long-term Yin deficiency), heat or fever in hands, feet and chest, a red narrow or thin tongue and a thready rapid pulse.

d) Blood Deficiency with Wind

Blood deficiency with wind can be diagnosed when observing spasms, tremors, palpitations, dizziness, fatigue, a red tongue and a thready and deficient pulse.

Treatment

Apply acupuncture to DU20, DU25, SP4, LI4, LI11, LIV14, LIV2 and UB18. Refer to the emergency treatment section in Chapter 10 for more information.

10) Cold Residing in the Liver Channel

Cause

Cold stagnation in the liver channel occurs from an external cold invasion.

Symptoms

Pain or cold sensation in the groin.

Swelling in groin area, cold sensation and a downward pulling sensation of the testes

Tongue will be pale (deficient people), white moist coat

Pulse will be slow, deep, wiry (cold, pain)

Treatment

To treat the problem, the liver channel must be warmed up and the cold must be dispersed. The underlying deficiency must also be tonified. Apply moxa to the LIV3, LIV8, LIV10, LIV11 and ST36.

Heart

The Heart is considered to hold the wisdom of the body. It is the emperor, master of circulation, the regulator and the house of the spirit. The tongue is the mirror of the heart, acting as the external sensor, the tip of the tongue in particular. If a person has a big tongue, then he or she probably has a big heart. For men the pulse on the right wrist will be weaker while for women, the pulse on the left wrist (where the heart pulse is located) will be weaker. The quality and condition of the heart is shown on the points between the eyebrows.

Although the lung is generally affected by sadness first, the heart can be directly effected by extreme sadness such as the death of a spouse: the internal effect will be directly on the heart, then the lung. This is why so many people will die shortly after the death of their spouse.

Men have heart attacks more often than women. This is mainly due to higher stress levels, poor diet, drinking or smoking. An impending heart attack will generally begin as palpitations. The patient notices overtime that he or she will become forgetful. They may have many dreams but not remember them. These dreams will eventually become nightmares or dreams where they see dead friends or relatives or may hear someone calling their name. Their bed or body may begin to shake and in some cases, they will see their own funeral. Koreans take spirits very seriously. In the countryside sounds travel far, especially on a foggy day. If someone hears their name called, they would wait for the three time before answering. This is because if a person with a weak heart answers the door on the first call and find nobody there, it could cause a serious heart condition.

Why do these things occur? The heart controls the spirit of the individual. As the heart becomes weaker, it is unable to defend against these unwanted spirits which is why these dreams occur. The elderly will often see spirits as their heart grows weaker. Women who embark on a fasting meditation are more likely to see spirits since their hearts are generally weaker than men's. These types of symptoms can also occur if the heart is restricted. People who sleep on their left side may experience an increase in nightmares because the heart, which is on the left side, becomes compressed. Since two-thirds of the heart is on the left side of the body, paralysis caused by heart problems will more often occur on the left side. Getting goose bumps after hearing voices, a stutter or insomnia may indicate a heart problem.

Medication which acts as muscle relaxer will often come with a warning of nightmares. Muscle relaxers relax the heart, weakening its ability to control the spirit.

There was a patient who once visited my office complaining of palpitations. He was about 30 years-old and athletic. When I checked his pulse, I immediately identified a heart problem due to a weak heart pulse. I began to treat him, and advised him to put his hands and feet in warm water whenever he felt the palpitations coming. During an eight-month period, he had three serious attacks of palpitations. The first two times, he panicked and called 911. The third time, he was able to remember my instructions and followed them through. In a matter of minutes, the palpitations went away and he was able to drive himself to the hospital. In the case of heart palpitations or attack, immediately put the patient's hands and feet in warm water.

A female patient came into my office recently asking if anything could be done for the insomnia and nightmares she was experiencing. She had visited a psychiatrist but there was nothing he could do. After checking her pulse and investigating her past, I discovered two things, she had a heart weakness and had recently been to a funeral. After a few treatments, the insomnia and nightmares went away. People with heart weakness should avoid going to funerals or cemeteries, otherwise a worsening of their condition may occur.

Often, nurses working in nursing homes will observe elderly and sick patients having conversations with apparently with no one. The same patients may also dream of dead friends and relatives. These phenomena are common to everyone with heart illness, chronic illness or just before death. Modern Western science denies that our spirit (Ling, Hun, Po) leaves our body after death or that one can be possessed by the spirit of a deceased person. How a person lived his or her life will determine whether the person will face a good or evil spirit upon death. This is true for all of us, regardless of whether or not we believe in eternity.

The following points are important points which can be treated with acupuncture when there is heart weakness. The location of these points are described in detail at the end of Chapter 10.

THE SPIRIT POINTS

UB15 Xin Shu

Heart's Hollows - This is the heart back shu point found next to the 5th thoracic vertebra.

REN14 Juque

Great Palace - This is the heart front mu point.

REN8 Shen que

Spirit's Palace - This point can be found at the center of the Umbilicus. No acupuncture should be applied here and indirect moxa only.

DU10 Ling tai

Spirit's Platform - This point is below the spinous process of the 6th Thoracic Vertebra.

DU11 Shen dao

Spirit's Path - Below the spinis process of the 5th Thoracic Vertebra.

DU24 Shen ting

Spirit's Hall - On the midsagillal line of the head, 0.5 cun within the hairline.

UB44 - Shen dang

This is known as the house of the spirit. It is found next to UB15, next to the scapula and should be treated for the bad dreams.

H7, Shen men

This is the spirit gate where spirits come and go.

K23, Shen feng

This is the spirit seal keeping spirits in or out.

K25, Shen cang

This is the where the spirit is stored.

UB42, Pofu

Known as the soul's household, it is located next to the 3rd thoracic vertebra next to the scapula.

UB47, Hun men

This is the soul's door.

H4, Ling dao

This point is located on the wrist and is known as the spirit's path.

K24, ling xu

Located at the 3rd intercostal space between REN and the nipple, it is the soul's ruins.

THE 13 GHOST POINTS

The body has what is known as ghost points. Both Sun Si-Miao and Guang Un San have written about these points and treatment methods to cure what is known in the West as possession. Korean and Chinese Taoists have had differing opinions regarding the nature of spirits but it is agreed that not all spirits are bad. Many people possessed by a good spirit become shamans or healers. This possession can take place at birth or during a person's lifetime. I do not treat this type of problem, however I can recommend a very good acupuncturist in China. Remember that a person who suffers from manic depression or schizophrenia should not be treated as if they were possessed by spirits. There is no basis for treating the ghost points of patient's whose problems are psychologically based.

To treat this problem, all thirteen points must receive strong stimulation beginning with P5 (see Figure 10-35). (Strong stimulation means to vibrate the needle frequently and to make the points hot by applying moxa.) The thirteen points are as follows (remember that P5 stimulation must come first):

1. REN26 - Ghost Palace

2. LU11 - Ghost Convincing

3. SP1 - Ghost Fortress

4. LU9 - Ghost Heart

5. UB62 - Ghost Road

6. DU14 - Ghost Pillow

7. DU 16 - Ghost Bed

8. REN24 - Ghost Market

9. PC8 - Ghost Cave

10. DU23 - Ghost Hall

11. REN1 - Ghost Hidden

12 LI11 - Ghost Minister

13. Under Tongue - Ghost Seal

1) HEART QI DEFICIENCY

CAUSE

Heart Qi deficiency may be as a result of chronic bleeding or chronic illness. Emotional problems such as irritation or sadness can depress heart Qi and spirit. A patient born with a weak heart or constitutional weakness may also have this syndrome.

SYMPTOMS

Symptoms will include palpitation, shortness of breath, a pale face, feeling tired and weak, spontaneous sweating or an unclear shen (spirit). The patient's pulse will be weak with an irregular beat and the tongue will be pale and flabby (edema) and swollen from a lack of circulation.

TREATMENT

Efforts must be made to tonify the heart and spleen Qi as well as pacify the shen. Acupuncture should be applied to REN14 (mu point), UB15 and REN17. To tonify the heart Qi, concentrate on P6, P4, REN6; to stimulate the heart beat rate and raise blood pressure, H5, DU25 (tip of nose); to decrease the heart beat rate, P5, P6, UB15, ST9, UB1, UB2, ST1; to control palpitations, P6, P4, UB15, REN14, H7, P6, REN6, UB20 and UB21.

2) HEART YANG DEFICIENCY

This type of deficiency is similar to Qi deficiency and cold. Kidney Yang deficiency caused by too much sex, work, or exposure to cold weather can become a heart Yang deficiency. Heart Qi deficiency allowed to continue over a long period of time will become heart Yang deficiency.

SYMPTOMS

Symptoms will include cold limbs, intolerance to cold, stuffiness in heart area, a bright pale face (edema) and shortness of breath aggravated by movement. The tongue will be blue in extreme cases, pale, flabby and damp. The pulse will be deep, weak, irregular and slow.

Other symptoms include:

Profuse sweating

Pulse is weak and fading

Fear (pain with palpitation)

Western symptom - coronary heart disease

TREATMENT

The Yang must be retrieved and the heart tonified. Apply acupuncture and moxa as follows:

H5 needle, REN6 and UB15 should receive moxa and needle, DU14 (all Yang channels meet)

If there is a chronic heart failure condition, then:

First Treatment - P6, P5, H8

Rotate - P6, P4, P3

Strengthen spleen - ST36, ST25, REN12

3) HEART BLOOD DEFICIENCY

CAUSE

This can be caused by a spleen deficiency, malnourishment or lack of absorption of nutrients. Emotional conditions such as anxiety can cause stress on the heart as well as bleeding or hemorrhaging.

SYMPTOMS

Pale face and lips

Fatigue

Nighttime palpitations

Daytime palpitations - Qi deficiency when occurs with activity

Insomnia - deficiency type is when the blood is unable to nourish the spirit. The patient will be restless and anxious.

The patient will experience dream disturbed sleep (nightmares).

Treatment

In this case, tonify heart, nourish blood and pacify shen by applying acupuncture to UB17 (blood), UB20 (spleen), UB23 (kidney), UB15 (heart), REN14, REN15, REN4, H7 and P6.

4) HEART YIN DEFICIENCY

CAUSE

This deficiency can be caused by kidney Yin deficiency resulting from too much work, sex, drugs, anxiety, worrying, stress or external heat which can injure the heart or the Yin of the body. Summer heat or exposure to high temperatures could injure the Yin of the body.

SYMPTOMS

Palpitations

Insomnia

Anxiety or restlessness

Night sweating

Afternoon fever

Malar flush

Irritability

Dryness of the mouth and throat

Poor memory

Distrust of other people

The tongue will be red with no coat and the pulse will be thready and rapid.

TREATMENT

Tonify heart, nourish heart Yin and calm the spirit. Apply acupuncture to H6, REN14, K6, REN4, REN7, SP6 nourish heart Yin, H7 and P6 to calm spirit, UB15, REN14, H7, P6 for anxiety; and H7, P6, SP6, UB23, UB15, K3 for insomnia.

5) Heart Fire Rising

Cause

This can be due to emotional problems (similar to liver fire rising), leading to irritation, worrying, Qi compression and possibly explosion. A liver fire rising condition can also lead to a heart fire.

Symptoms

Thirsty, headache

Dark urine

Pain with urination

Blood in urine

Feel warm or hot, red face

Insomnia

Red tongue with yellow coat, sometimes showing ulcerated tip

Pulse will be rapid and full or large

The patient may also have a bitter taste in the mouth. If this happens in the morning, then there is heart fire. If it occurs all day, then there is liver fire.

In more severe cases, the heart fire may invade the small intestine which in turn invades the urinary bladder causing painful urination. Often liver fire and heart fire occur together. The heart should be treated first.

Treatment

Disperse fire and pacify the shen by applying acupuncture to H8 (to draw out heat), H9 and UB15. To tonify and nourish heart Yin; REN14, REN15, SP6, K6, H7.

6) Heart Blood Stagnation

This is generally caused by heart Qi or Yang deficiency. If the condition is chronic, then the blood can become stagnant and Qi deficiency with cold could cause heart blood stagnation. It may also be due to emotional problems such as excess anxiety, resentment, anger or grief. These problems tend to disturb the spirit.

SYMPTOMS

Pain in the heart region

Pricking, stabbing pain

Shooting pain from shoulder and back down the arm through small intestine channel

Weakness and shortness of breath

Stuffiness in the heart

Pale and bluish color on lips and finger nails

The tongue will be reddish on tip with purplish spots and the pulse will be slow, choppy, and thready with a missed beat.

Western symptoms will include coronary artery disease, angina pectoralis, cardiac insufficiency and palpitations.

TREATMENT

The blood must be activated and the coagulation dispersed. If deficiency exists, tonify Qi and Yang. If strong emotions are involved, use herbs.

Apply acupuncture to SP10, UB17 to move blood; REN17, H6, P6, P4 and asi points for chest pains; and H7, P6, UB15, REN14 for emotional problems.

7) PHLEGM MISTING THE HEART

CAUSE

Consumption of too much greasy food and alcohol will cause adult spleen dysfunction. A child jing deficiency is a constitutional weakness. Many overweight people will have misting heart condition with coronary disease.

SYMPTOMS

Mental confusion

Difficult to speak

Stutter

Nausea, vomiting

Coma (phlegm plugs up the orifice of heart or rattling phlegm in throat)

Pain in chest, left arm

Coronary artery disease

Cough with a lot of phlegm

No appetite

A child with this syndrome may have mental retardation. An adult may fall into a coma induced by a stroke.

The tongue will be sticky with a greasy white coat or yellow if there is heat. The pulse is slippery, fast or slow and has a smooth or gliding quality.

TREATMENT

Resolve phlegm, open orifice and remove the heat. Acupuncture ST40, REN12, UB20 (spleen), H5, P7, H9 (tonify and open heart).

8) PHLEGM FIRE AGITATING THE HEART

CAUSE

Severe emotional problems can cause this problem. Compressed Qi transforms to fire (or eating too much cold greasy food). It can also be caused by heat invasion from outside (summer heat). This condition will affect the heart and pericardium.

SYMPTOMS

Palpitation

Stabbing chest pain

Red face

Desire for cold drinks

Anger

Insomnia and sleep with many dreams or nightmares

Coma

Nose bleeds

Blood in urine

There may also be mental confusion, irrational behavior, shouting, incoherent speech and crying or laughing without cause. The tongue will be red with a thick yellow greasy coat and the pulse will be slippery or wiry and rapid.

TREATMENT

Clear the fire, resolve and dispel the phlegm and pacify the spirit. Acupuncture UB15 and REN14, ST40 (sedate) for the phlegm, UB20, SP6 & REN12 to tonify, and to clear the fire, LIV3 & LIV2 (sedate), H9 and H8. To resolve the phlegm, treat P7, P9, P5. Herbs also work well.

SPLEEN

Western medicine believes that the spleen's main function is to remove old or defective blood cells and platelets and filter out foreign matter in the blood. Eastern medicine believes that the spleen manages the transformation and transportation of food to produce Qi and blood. In doing so, it plays a major role in keeping the organs in place, preventing organ prolapse or a hernia. It helps to develop strong muscles, control blood production and menstruation. A deficient spleen will result in a patient being bruised easily and often the patient's mouth will remain slightly open.

The spleen is the storehouse for reasoning, understanding, ideas and opinions. Spleen Qi deficiency will cause a poor appetite, pale lips and cause the person to think or worry too much resulting in emotional problems.

The stomach and spleen are closely related. The stomach likes moisture whereas the spleen likes dryness. If reversed, the spleen will cause dampness and the stomach will cause stagnation. If the Qi rises, vomiting will be the result. If the Qi goes down, the result is diarrhea. Water temperature can disrupt the spleen. A baby should always been given water at room temperature. Cold drinks such as water or milk may inhibit the growth of a child as well as causing the child to be under weight. An adult should also avoid cold drinks but unlike a child, cold water causes an adult to gain weight. Essentially, the body is tricked into thinking it is winter and as a result will take on more weight. Regardless of whether the person is a child or an adult, cold drinks will cause a dampness condition.

1) SPLEEN QI DEFICIENCY

CAUSES

Spleen Qi deficiency can often be the result of poor eating habits. Typically, consumption of cold food, too much or too little food can bring Spleen Qi deficiency. Generally, it begins as liver Qi weakness. Liver Qi affects the stomach Qi which in turn affects the spleen Qi. Chronic conditions of the heart, lung or spleen may also bring about a spleen Qi deficiency problem. Other causes can be a lack of exercise or a constitutional weakness.

A pure vegetarian diet will also cause a spleen Qi deficiency. Consuming animal protein helps to tonify the spleen and blood.

SYMPTOMS

Symptoms include fatigue, weakness in the limbs and muscles (muscular atrophy), a dull or pale complexion, swelling and distention of the abdomen, loose stool, dizziness (from a lack of blood and nourishment), lack of appetite and nausea or gas in the stomach. Often, the pain in the stomach is relieved when the stomach is touched or pressed on. The tongue will be pale, flabby with teeth marks and the pulse will be weak and thready.

TREATMENT

Steps to strengthen the spleen and tonify the Qi must be taken. Acupuncture on REN12 for the stomach and UB20 for the spleen will help. Also, apply acupuncture to ST36 to tonify and strengthen the digestion and P6 to control abdominal region and to stop any nausea or vomiting. SP4, ST25, LIV13 and ST40 are the additional points to focus on.

If the patient vomits after eating, apply moxa to ST36, P6, REN12, SP4 and UB20. Moxa is effective for Qi deficiency and fighting dampness.

2) SPLEEN QI SINKING

CAUSE

Spleen Qi sinking is caused by a chronic Qi deficiency where the organs have become depleted. Eating large amounts of food too quickly and without resting or going back to work too quickly will cause this syndrome.

SYMPTOMS

Symptoms include a prolapse of the stomach, uterus and anus. This often brings on hemorrhoids or chronic diarrhea.

TREATMENT

Treat this problem by tonifying the spleen Qi and raising the Yang Qi. To treat stomach prolapse, apply acupuncture to ST21 and ST25, DU20 (moxa or needle to tonify the Qi), ST36, REN12 and REN6. Abdominal exercises, eating smaller quantities of food and rest are also required.

To treat uterine prolapse, apply acupuncture to ST30 to invigorate and to GB28, SP6, DU20 and REN6 to tonify the Qi. Warm the needles on UB10, UB11, UB17, UB18, UB22, ST20, and ST21.

To treat anus prolapse, DU1, UB40, UB57, DU20 (moxa).

3) SPLEEN UNABLE TO GOVERN BLOOD

This is very similar to spleen Qi sinking. It is a chronic disease and/or spleen Qi deficiency.

SYMPTOMS

The patient will have a pale face, digestive problems, breathing problems, weak extremities, aversion to talking, blood in stool and urine or uterine bleeding. The tongue will be pale and the pulse will be weak and small. The patient will tend to bruise easily.

TREATMENT

Efforts must be made to tonify the spleen and retain blood in vessels. Acupuncture the blood point at UB17 and SP10. Tonify the spleen at ST36, SP6, REN6 and SP1.

Uterine bleeding can be caused by spleen Qi deficiency. There may be excessive bleeding which will be dark or pale in color and the patient may be cold and weak. Apply moxa to REN4, SP1,DU20 andTW4. Alternatively, you can apply acupuncture to UB20, UB18, SP6, SP1, REN4 and moxa to DU4.

4) Spleen Yang Deficiency

Cause

This deficiency can be caused by eating too many cold, greasy, raw or sweet foods over a long period of time. A long illness causing kidney Yang deficiency can lead to spleen Yang deficiency as well. Improper medication or overuse of Yin tonification will cause cooling which over a long period of time could deplete the digestive system.

Symptom

Qi deficiency cold

Watery stool (diarrhea)

Undigested food in the stool

Early morning diarrhea

Cold extremities

Dislike of cold weather

Eepigastric region pain

Relief from pain when treated with moxa

Fatigue

Edema

Pale face

Urination difficulties and a lack of appetite

The tongue will be pale, swollen with teeth marks and moist. The pulse will be weak, deep and slow.

Treatment

Attempts should be made to warm up the stomach area, tonify the spleen Qi and tonify the kidney Qi if it is deficient. Moxa should be applied to ST25, UB25, ST36, UB20, LIV13, SP3 and REN12.

5) Dampness Distressing The Spleen

Cause

This can be caused by spleen Qi deficiency and Yang deficiency leading to excess symptoms.

Symptoms

Typically, the patient will decrease food intake or feel a lack of appetite, have a fullness in the stomach, greasy, sticky sensation in the mouth, feel heavy, fatigued, edema and swelling, have a disturbed water metabolism and loose stool. The tongue will have a thick greasy white coat and the pulse will be slippery and soft.

Treatment

The spleen must be tonified and the dampness must be eliminated. The herbal formula will help to achieve this. Acupuncture can be applied to UB20, UB23, REN9 (moxa for deficiency condition) REN6 to tonify the Qi and SP6, ST36, ST40 and UB39.

6) Cold Damp Invading Spleen

Cause

This is an external acute condition brought about by eating too many cold foods such as ice cream, watermelon, cold drinks or raw greasy foods and/or by eating too quickly. Prolonged exposure to cold or rainy conditions can also cause cold damp invading spleen.

Symptoms

Symptoms are usually lack of appetite or feeling full, feeling tired, diarrhea, cold abdominal pain, sensitive to being touched, comforted by heat (moxa), heavy feeling in the head and a sticky sweet taste in the mouth. The tongue will be greasy with a white coat and the pulse will be soft and slippery.

Treatment

The cold dampness must be dispersed. The stomach must be warmed and the spleen tonified. Apply acupuncture to ST25, ST40, UB20, SP3, UB25, ST36, LIV13 and REN12.

7) Spleen Stomach Damp Heat

Cause

In this case, the spleen is attacked by heat. A hot or humid climate can bring this on. Consumption of too much alcohol, smoking and greasy spicy foods can also result in spleen stomach damp heat.

Symptoms

The patient may have a yellowish tinge on the skin or eyes (jaundice). He may feel congested in the chest, have abdominal distention, nausea, vomiting, bitter taste or poor appetite, dark yellow urine and constipation or diarrhea. The tongue will have a thick yellow greasy coat and the pulse will be rapid, slippery or soft.

Western symptoms may be glomerulonephritis, either acute or chronic with a slight fever, cloudy incontinent urination (bladder infection) or infectious hepatitis.

Treatment

The heat must be cooled and the dampness dispersed.

Cold Damp (For Reference)

Cold damp is typically marked by diarrhea, a watery stool, intolerance to cold, lack of thirst, a pale tongue and a slow deep pulse. Apply acupuncture to ST25, UB25, ST36, REN12, SP9, REN6 and LI4.

The patient may have dysentery which can be diagnosed if the patient has scanty stools, white mucus, dull pain, no thirst, tastelessness, a white greasy tongue and a deep slow pulse.

Damp Heat

Damp heat is also marked by diarrhea but this will be yellow, hot and foul smelling. There will be a burning sensation in the anus, abdominal pain, aversion to heat and yellow scanty urine. The tongue will be yellow and greasy and the pulse will be rapid and slippery. Treat this by applying acupuncture to ST25, UB25, ST36, LI4, ST44 and SP9.

If a patient has dysentery, it will be difficult to move bowels, there will be abdominal pain, red and white mucus in the stool, fever, nausea and vomiting. The tongue will be yellow and greasy and the pulse will be rapid.

8) STOMACH FIRE BLAZING

CAUSE

The typical cause of this ailment is excess heat in the stomach caused by eating too many hot spicy foods. Overwork may also cause this condition.

SYMPTOMS

Typically, the patient will display swollen and/or bleeding gums, abdominal pain, bad breath, excessive appetite and thirst, a burning sensation in the epigastiric area, a red tongue with a yellow coat and a full, large and rapid pulse.

TREATMENT

The patient should have the fire cooled and the stomach nourished. Acupuncture ST44, ST43, ST36, UB21 and REN12.

9) STOMACH YIN DEFICIENCY

CAUSE

This is caused by long term chronic dehydration where the patient does not drink enough fluids. In general, Yin deficiency can be caused by anxiety or overwork.

SYMPTOMS

The patient will exhibit a dry mouth and lip condition, constipation due to a lack of fluid in the digestive system, nausea, feeling the need to vomit but cannot, belching, no appetite and irritability. There may also be malar flush, insomnia, night sweats and heat on palms and soles of feet. The tongue will be red with cracks and have no coat and the pulse will be thready and rapid.

TREATMENT

To treat this, nourish the Yin and soothe and moisten the stomach with acupuncture to SP6, K3, P6, REN12, UB21, ST36 and LI11.

10) STOMACH FOOD STAGNATION

CAUSE

This occurs when the patient has eaten too much greasy food or eats irregularly. Generally, there is a weak stomach condition where the patient is unable to digest. The tongue will have a thick greasy coat and the pulse will be slippery indicating retention.

SYMPTOMS

The patient will experience bloating, stomach aches, nausea, vomiting, lack of appetite and diarrhea or constipation. In general, the Western term that comes closest to this condition is indigestion.

TREATMENT

Acupuncture REN12, ST 25, ST36, ST44, LIV13 and P6.

LUNG

The lung is the manager and master of the Qi and respiration. The lung is the defensive system maintaining the order and rhythm of the body as well as the water metabolism. It moistens the skin and hair and controls the pores for sweating. The lung opens to the nose. Sadness and grief will effect the lung directly but if the sadness is extreme such as the death of a spouse, the internal effect will be first on the heart, then the lung.

Lung disorders can result from irregular life patterns, which cause stress on the lung functions. Dryness and cold or a change of seasons will also cause lung conditions. Energy will be depleted as lungs become weaker. The lung conditions are symbolized by a superficial pulse, crying, grief, sadness and a desire for pungent or spicy foods. The lung conditions will be worse around mid-day and start to get better as the afternoon comes. The patient may also wake up at 3 to 5 a.m. A runny nose is usually a result of fluid coming from the lung. Short-term illness may be the result of lung Qi deficiency. Smoke, chemicals and dust can bring about a lung imbalance.

A white male patient 30 years of age had been on a vegetarian diet for many years. During that time, his weight dropped from 210 pounds to 175 pounds. He had a severe Yang deficiency and no libido. He had several lung related ailments including bronchitis and psoriasis (dermatitis). His wife stopped into my clinic and I gave her herbs for Yang tonification and to moisten the lungs and told her to make sure her husband started to eat meat. Shortly after, his illness was cured. A short while later, his psoriasis came back. I discovered that he had taken a trip to Arizona where the air is very dry.

In another case, a sixty year-old woman had stopped smoking after 30 years. She suffered from skin rashes, fatigue and dry skin and hair. These are all symptoms of lung deficiency. Her symptoms were compounded by deep sadness after attending a funeral.

1) LUNG QI DEFICIENCY

CAUSE

This deficiency is the result of stress and prolonged disease. Environmental stresses such as smog is a common cause.

SYMPTOMS

Coughing, shortness of breath, weak or low voice, not talkative, pale facial color and a lack of natural warmth, either physical or mental, are typical symptoms. The patient may also experience spontaneous perspiration during the day, become easily exhausted and catch colds easily. There will also be a thin clear sputum and the tongue will be pale, thin and have a white coat. The pulse will be weak.

TREATMENT

The lung Qi must be tonified. Acupuncture UB13, LU1, LU9, LU7, ST36, REN6, REN17 and UB43.

2) LUNG YIN DEFICIENCY

CAUSE

This is an excess deficiency where the patient may become susceptible to chronic lung disease. Continually breathing of dry air, smoking, living in the desert or working in a dry environment can also cause this deficiency.

SYMPTOMS

Dry cough (hacking), dry throat or a coarse voice and afternoon fever should be expected. The patient may feel as if steaming heat is coming from the bones. There may be fever, night sweats, hot flashes in the evening and heat in the chest. The tongue will be red and thin with no coat and the pulse will be thready and rapid. Western physicians who examine a patient with these conditions might diagnose pneumonia or tuberculosis.

TREATMENT

Nourish the Yin and moisten and lubricate the lung. Apply acupuncture to LU6, DU14, UB13, ST36, LU1, UB17, H6, H7 and LU9. You can also treat SP6 and K3 for Yin tonification.

3) WIND COLD ATTACKING THE LUNGS - COLD INVADING THE LUNGS

SYMPTOMS

This is a typically also known as a cold. It will be accompanied by chills and fever, runny nose, white sputum, headaches, nasal obstruction, no perspiration, itchy throat, coughing, shortness of breath, asthma and dyspnea. The pulse will be superficial and tight and the tongue will have a thin white coat.

TREATMENT

The lungs need to be warmed up, the lung Qi needs to be expanded. Apply moxa or acupuncture to DU16, GB20, UB12 LI4, K7, LU7, UB13 and LU5.

4) WIND HEAT ATTACKING THE LUNGS

SYMPTOMS

When this occurs, there will be heat damage to the Yin. There may also be a fever, intolerance to wind and heat, nasal discharge (thick and yellow), thirst, sore throat, constipation, dark urine, sweating, nose bleeds and chronic asthma or dyspnea and shortness of breath. The tongue will have a thin yellow coat and the tip will be red. The pulse will be superficial and rapid.

TREATMENT

The heat must be cleared and the lung nourished. Acupuncture DU14 to reduce the heat, TW5 and GB20 to clear the wind heat, LU11 to relieve exterior and dispel heat and LU5, UB13 and LU7 for the cough.

5) PHLEGM DAMPNESS IN THE LUNGS

CAUSE

This is due to external dampness. There may have been rapid cooling of the body or the patient may have been eating cold raw food over a long period of time. This will disturb the water metabolism which could cause spleen deficiency.

SYMPTOMS

Phlegm may be obstructing the passage of Qi. There will be shortness of breath, profuse sputum, profuse phlegm with bubbles. The breathing difficulty may become more severe when lying down. The chest will also feel congested. The tongue will have a greasy coat. If the coat is yellow, then there is heat. If it is white, then there is cold. The patient may also have difficulty sleeping at night.

If the lung has been invaded by a liver problem, the patient will experience a cough plus pain in the ribs. There will be a bitter taste in the mouth, irritability, stress and emotional problems.

TREATMENT

Acupuncture to UB20, LI4, and ST40. Treat DU14, LU11, L7 (lung Qi) and LU5 (cough) for phlegm heat. REN22, REN21, REN17, ST40, REN4, ST36, LI4, UB12 and UB13 for asthma and acute wheezing.

6) LUNG DRYNESS AND HEAT

This is a typical summer and early autumn problem.

SYMPTOMS

The patient will find it difficult to expectorate. The nasal passage and throat will be dry. The tongue will be dry, have a red tip and a thin yellow coat. The pulse will be superficial and rapid.

TREATMENT

The dryness must be lubricated and the lungs must be cleared of phlegm. Also, the spleen and lung Qi should be tonified. Apply acupuncture to LU1, UB13 and LU6 to disperse heat. LU5 for the cough, SP6, K3, DU14 and LI4.

LARGE INTESTINE

1) LARGE INTESTINE DAMP HEAT

CAUSE

This is brought on by consumption of too much alcohol, too much greasy food or improper diet, damp heat, stagnation of food or a bladder infection.

SYMPTOMS

The patient will often feel an urgent need for bowel movements and there will be a burning sensation in the anus. There may also be blood, white mucus and a foul smell. Lower abdominal pain will intensify after bowel movements. The tongue will be greasy, have a yellow coat and appear red. The pulse will be slippery and rapid.

TREATMENT

The dampness must be dispelled and the heat cleared. Apply acupuncture to ST25, ST36, LI4, LI11, ST44, UB 25 and SP9.

2) LARGE INTESTINE DRIES UP

SYMPTOMS

The patient will have constipation, Yin deficiency and fluid deficiency. The tongue will be red and dry and the pulse will be thready and rapid.

TREATMENT

Treat the following points with acupuncture: TW6, ST25, ST36, REN12, K6, SP6, ST37 and UB 25.

KIDNEY

The kidney is associated with the cold or winter. It is also associated with salt, blackness and fear, mourning and growing voices in the Five Element Theory.

Jing (essence) is the Yin aspect of the kidney. It is the storehouse for vital essence. The actions of hormones, growth, reproduction, puberty and menopause can be traced to the kidney.

Jing creates bone marrow, the spine, the brain and develops mentality. For problems in the uterus, fertility, a child's growth, bone and teeth, manufacture of blood, hair or hearing, look towards the kidney because these are all related to the jing.

The kidney is the ruler of the water metabolism. Edema problems result from an unhealthy kidney. Kidney Yang steams and moistens the body. A kidney Yang deficiency will result in lung problems and frequent urination. The kidney controls the absorption of water from the lung.

The kidney is also the receptacle of Qi. Qi comes from the lungs and is maintained in the Kidney. The ear is the external opening of the kidney.

1) KIDNEY YIN DEFICIENCY

CAUSE

The Kidney Yin deficiency can be the result of overwork, chronic illness, anxiety, stress, too much sex, drug abuse, dehydration, blood loss due to injury, post surgery (lack of appetite), overuse of Yang tonic (herbs) or chronic illness.

SYMPTOMS

Ear ringing, dizziness, night sweating, constipation, dark urine, dry mouth or throat are typical symptoms of kidney Yin deficiency. There may be a tidal fever in the palms, feet or chest. Also poor memory, sore lower back, deafness and nocturnal emissions during dreams with orgasm. The tongue will be red, no coat and have cracks. The pulse will be thready and rapid.

TREATMENT

The Yin needs to be tonified and the kidney should be nourished. Apply acupuncture to REN4, K3, K10, SP6, K9, DU14, UB23 and DU20. American ginseng is good for kidney Yin deficiency.

2) KIDNEY YANG DEFICIENCY

CAUSE

This can be caused by too much sex, excess emotions, overwork, coldness, chronic disease, poor diet or old age.

SYMPTOMS

Lower back pain

Impotency

Premature ejaculation

Infertility

Abundant clear urine

Scanty clear urine (severe case)

Edema in the leg

Early morning diarrhea

Watery stools with undigested food

Weak legs and knees

Nocturnal emissions without orgasm during dreams

Bright white pale face

Fatigue

Dislike of cold

Cold extremities

No energy

Poor appetite

Perspiration after a little exertion

Like to sleep a lot

Sleep a lot but always tired

Libido is very low

The pulse will be deep, weak and slow and the tongue will be pale, swollen, moist and have teeth marks.

TREATMENT

To treat kidney Yang deficiency, tonify Yang and kidney by applying acupuncture to REN4, DU4, REN6, UB23, K7, UB52, ST36 and SP6. For edema, UB39 and use moxa on REN9 to increase urination. For dampness excess, SP9 and ST28. These points will need strong stimulation.

3) KIDNEY QI DEFICIENCY

CAUSE

Kidney Qi deficiency is a Yin and Yang deficiency. There will be Qi weakness but no false heat or coldness. It can be caused by:

Excess sex

Chronic disease

Getting old too fast

Over work (standing or lifting objects)

Constitutional weakness

SYMPTOMS

The patient will experience:

Urinary problems and lower back pain

Frequent urination at night

Clear urine, profuse (lack of control) or dribbling

Premature ejaculation

Seminal emission

Fatigue, weakness

Cold extremities

Shortness of breath

Tongue will be pale and the pulse will be weak.

TREATMENT

Tonify the Qi and the kidney. Acupuncture treatment is the same as kidney Yang deficiency where treatment of REN4, REN6, DU4, UB23, UB52 is called for. Also, UB58 and UB60 for lower back weakness and pain, UB28 for frequent urination (use ginger moxa[41] on UB28 and UB23), REN9 and UB39 for edema and K4 and K7 to tonify the kidney.

4) Kidney Jing Deficiency

Jing is the Yin quality and the congenital aspect of growth, development and reproduction. In children, it determines growth and development and could be the cause of any mental or physical problems. As the person gets older, it affects the hormone, aging, puberty and menopause.

Symptoms

Difficulty inhaling

Perspire easily

Difficulty with menstrual cycle

Hormonal imbalance

Night sweating

Malar flush (cheek bone)

Restlessness

Old age symptoms such as

- Loss of hair

- Senility

- Rapid degeneration of body

Constitutional problems like

- Bended back

- Under development of bone, tendons

- Under development of mental abilities

Sexual impotency

Tooth decay

Insomnia

The pulse will be thready and not rapid and the tongue will be red without a coat.

Treatment

The kidney, jing, Yin and Yang must be tonified. Acupuncture should be applied to UB23, UB52, DU4, K3, REN6 and DU20.

Yin Deficinet Symptoms of Each Organ

++ MORE   + YES   - NO   +- SOMETIMES

	HEART	KIDNEY	LIVER	ST/SP	LUNG
Palpitation	+	-	-	-	-
Dry Cough	-	-	-	-	+
Sticky Bloody Sputum	-	-	-	-	+
Hoarse Voice	-	-	-	-	+-
Anorexia, Nausea	-	-	-	+	-
Nocturnal Emission or Irregular Menses	-	+	+	-	-
Dizziness	-	+	+	-	-
Dry Eyes	-	-	+	-	-
Tinnitus	-	+	+	-	-
Poor Memory	+	+	+	-	-
Insomnia	+	+	+	-	-

Table 12-1

Yang Deficinet Symptoms of Each Organ

++ MORE   + YES   - NO   +- SOMETIMES

	HEART	KIDNEY	LIVER	SPLEEN	LUNG
Palpitation	+	-	-	-	-
Shortness of Breath	+	+	-	-	+
Cold Extremities	+-	++	-	+	-
Edema	+-	++	-	+	+-
Sex (Low)	-	+	-	-	-
Poor Appetite	-	-	-	+	-
Loose Stool	-	+	-	++	-
Cough	-	-	-	-	+
Chest pain	+	-	-	-	+-
Tongue	Pale, Sometimes with Purple Spots	Pale	-	Pale with teeth marks	Pale
Pulse	Thready, Missed Beat	Kidney position weak	-	Soft	Thready

Table 12-2

* The liver does not have Yang deficiency symptoms. Liver problems will always be Yang and fire rising up conditions or a Yin deficiency or false heat symptoms with anger.

CONCLUSION

In this chapter, all disease patterns are categorized separately. But in reality, a patient's disease can vary in degree of severity and may also be the result of many syndromes. A patient can also have physical injuries and surgical scars which block acupuncture channels as described in Chapter 10. In most cases, a patient will display a combination of internal and external problems. Even emotional problems cause disease. Whether the practitioners of Oriental Medicine like it or not, they will be faced with patients who bring Western medical diagnosis and terms to them.

A woman patient came to my office complaining of many symptoms such as lethargy, heart palpitations, digestive problems and insomnia, as well as phobias for which she was seeing a psychiatrist. She said that her blood pressure was 60/90 but an electrocardiogram did not show any abnormal heart rhythm. The diagnosis of Western medicine had concluded that her condition was simply

low blood pressure. But my Oriental medical diagnosis found that she had spleen dampness syndrome which was resulting in nausea and heavy feeling. She also had a heart Qi deficiency resulting in severe nightmares. She had to sleep with the light on every night. She also had gall bladder channel problems which were affecting the left side of her body. It seemed to me that she was possessed by spirits. I treated her with acupuncture, herbal medicine and Qi Gong instruction. Her condition improved within a month. She could sleep without a night light for the first time in ten years and her nausea and heart palpitations had almost completely disappeared. Her health dramatically improved just as her family was considering whether or not to take her to a mental institution.

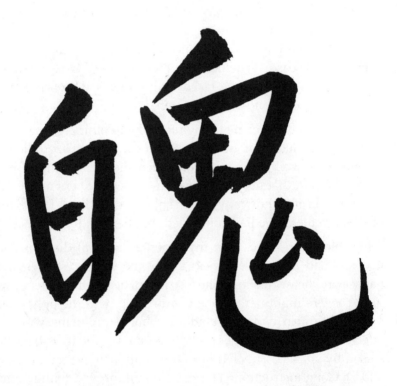

Po

Chapter 13

The Future of Oriental Medicine

A 35 year-old man who was otherwise in good health suffered an inguinal hernia. He went to an American acupuncturist who had been trained by a Chinese acupuncturist. The American acupuncturist treated the spleen channel of the patient according to the traditional Chinese method, but a hernia caused by a spleen Qi deficiency is usually found in the very old and weak or in a patient with a chronic illness. Most likely this American patient injured his lumbar area by an accident or had a sports injury that radiated pain and caused a Qi blockage to the Dai channel via the Gall Bladder channel. Another possibility is he was dating a woman and they:

(1) First had a nice dinner together, (2) went to a movie together, (3) listened to music together, (4) had a good conversation, (5) went to bed for sex. Perhaps he skipped 2, 3 and 4 as many young Americans do these days. Sex immediately after eating can cause a hernia due to the tension of a full stomach being pulled downward. Lunch time at his job is a half an hour. He may have to lift heavy objects or endure tremendous mental stress. Lifestyles in America or modern societies are much more complicated than those of Chinese people.

As I mentioned earlier in Chapter 11, Chinese people will get Carpal Tunnel Syndrome usually from malnutrition, Qi deficiency, or sprained or strained wrist joints, tendons or ligaments caused by heavy farming labor or factory work. American people usually get this syndrome from neck injuries caused by automobile accidents, sports injuries or bad posture during long hours of office work.

Medical researchers have found that the first generation of Korean emigrants in the U.S. had much less high blood pressure and high cholesterol levels and far fewer incidents of heart attacks than Americans. The second and third generations of Korean emigrants had the same rate of high blood pressure, high cholesterol and heart attacks as Americans since they shared the same levels of mental stress and consumed similar high levels of meat and fatty foods. This pattern was also observed in Chinese, Japanese and other Asian emigrants.

Asian women's breast cancer rate is much lower than that of American women. But recent surveys have found that Asian women living in the U.S. for more than ten years will become "Americanized" and will have the same breast cancer rate as American women.

An old and experienced Doctor of Oriental Medicine visiting the U.S. to treat his countrymen will treat their sickness as he would treat patients in his own country. It may be appropriate for the first generation of emigrants but the second and third generations are more Americanized. Therefore the diagnosis and treatment method must be changed to fit the lifestyles of Americans. The Oriental will have difficulty adjusting to this concept.

THE HISTORY OF ORIENTAL MEDICINE IN THE WEST AND U.S.

Oriental Medicine was first introduced to the Western world by Jesuits led by Matteo Ricci who lived in Macao, China in 1582. The first work in a European language about acupuncture was by the French Jesuit P.P. Harvieu, published in 1671. Eventually, it spread throughout Europe. There are approximately 60,000 medical doctors and 30,000 acupuncturists practicing in Europe today.

I moved to the United States from Korea in 1970 and published the book, "Acupuncture For Self Defense" in 1971. This book is out of print today but a revised edition will be published soon. It is known that the editor of *The New York Times*, James Reston, traveled with President Nixon to mainland China where he had an appendectomy with only acupuncture anesthesia. Since then, acupuncture treatment has become popular in the United States. Today, there are more than thirty states that license acupuncturists. Licensing is controlled by the National Commission for the Certification of Acupuncturists (N.C.C.A.) which was formed in 1982. The first acupuncture license exam was held in 1985. Besides the N.C.C.A. exam, each state has its own rules and regulations for licensing acupuncturists and Oriental herbalists. In California and Nevada, where the two medicines are combined and referred to as Oriental Medicine, only one license is issued. Other states require separate licenses or require a license for acupuncture only and no license for herbal medicine. The State of Massachusetts will require a license for Oriental herbal medicine until January of 1998. There are about 3,000 state-licensed acupuncturists and about 1,000 students in 30 acupuncture and Oriental Medicine schools in the United States today. But at the moment, the financial future of these graduates is not bright even after they get their licenses. That is because about 4,000 medical doctors practice acupuncture at the present time, most of whom do not have standard education in Oriental Medicine.

Western style pharmacists wanted to sell Oriental herbs at their stores. This angered licensed herbalists and doctors of Oriental Medicine. Both Eastern and Western medicine pharmacists protested against the practice for a year. Finally, the Health Ministry of the Korean Government decided that anyone who wanted to practice two medicines should graduate from both colleges of medicine and pass licensing exams in both fields.

In China, Korea and Japan four to six years of college are required for a license in Oriental Medicine and five to eight years of college is required for a license in Western medicine. The practice of both medicines requires national licenses in both fields. I think that this rule should be applied to United States and other countries as well. There are many non-licensed acupuncturists in Asian communities in the United States, about 100 times more than licensed acupuncturists. To make matters worse, they sometimes interview with local newspapers and present themselves as medicine men or shamen and give the false impression that colleges or licenses for Oriental Medicine do not exist in Asian countries. They generally charge much lower fees than licensed acupuncturists, treating Asians and some Americans. They open herbal medicine shops and decide that they have enough knowledge of Oriental Medicine to try and give acupuncture too. If you have been treated by an unqualified practitioner, you should check with the state board to inquire about the state's regulations on Oriental Medicine. If an herbal medicine shop prescribes herbs for Medicinal teas, check the doctor's background and license. He or she may mix your herbal tea with cheap tranquilizers, hormone pills or even antibiotics. It is safer to get raw herbs and brew them yourself or purchase them from an established company. Check whether the doctor washes his hands between patients and uses disposable paper towels. Does he or she have an autoclave for sterilization? If the doctor claims to use disposable needles, does he or she open each needle pack every time? Does the doctor purchase a fair amount of acupuncture needles every month or year? If you feel you have been treated by a careless and unqualified person, you should have your blood tested for AIDS, hepatitis and other viruses.

In rural areas in mainland China a barefoot doctor usually does not carry alcohol or other sterilization devices. The doctor may use many acupuncture needles, clean them by rubbing them with papers, and then reuse them. A barefoot doctor is a six-month or one-year trained acupuncturist for country or mountain people in mainland China.

Even if a doctor has an acupuncture license in the state where he or she practices acupuncture or herbal medicine, you should be able to communicate with him or her easily. Ask a few simple questions about basic biology, anatomy and physiology such as "What is the difference between bacteria and viruses?"

In Asian countries or in the United States, the news media may occasionally feature an old herbalist or Doctor of Oriental Medicine. Suddenly the person's business becomes prosperous and many patients are treated. If this person is not fully qualified, the herbalist Qi becomes depleted when performing acupuncture and anxieties over non-licensed practice can cause further Qi stagnation. This could result in the Qi stagnation of patients. Eventually the non-licensed acupuncturist shortens his or her life by Qi depletion and stagnation.

"One who deals with Qi and healing art whether he recognizes the flow of Qi or not, should be pure in his body and soul." Myung Kim.

Use your common sense and judgment when you visit Oriental herb shops and acupuncturists. Check their license and their background. Sometimes the practitioners speaks fluent English but their main study in college was not Oriental Medicine. When you choose a doctor check around. It is one of the most important decisions to make in your lifetime, so choose a doctor as you would a good friend or spouse. A bad relationship with a friend or spouse can be broken and recovered from but a bad medical treatment cannot be easily corrected by other treatment.

The FDA (United States Food and Drug Administration), and state and city health departments need to educate Asian communities on acupuncture sanitation. Otherwise, this country, already known as the AIDS kingdom, will become the United States of hepatitis and AIDS.

Most medical practitioners are required to maintain a high level of expertise through continuing education in order to renew their license. If complaints are registered or improprieties are discovered, their license may be suspended or revoked. Neighborhood herbalists, on the other hand, are not monitored.

You should check the background of the one who checks your pulse and palpates your body and asks many questions on your health and diseases. As with all health professionals, there may have been criminal or sexual charges against practitioners.

Some state regulations require that a patient sees a medical doctor or dentist to get a referral for acupuncture treatment. Is it really necessary?

Occasionally, these doctors may treat patients with acupuncture and herbal medicine themselves, ignoring the rights of Oriental Medicine practitioners. But what about the rights of their patients? Patients should not be treated like test animals in a lab.

A woman visited my clinic with cancer of the liver. Unfortunately, even after surgery on her breast and ovarian cancer, it had metastasized on her lung and liver. I could not help her much. There was no hope and she died a few months later. Upon my examination, I found out that she had a long history of lower back pain, sciatic pain and gall bladder channel problems. She had been treated by an Asian herbalist who had no license for medicine but had a business license and an Acupuncture Association Membership Certificate on the wall. This person prescribed herbal medicine for three years without knowing that her cancer was a result of problems with the gall bladder channel.

In Japan today, there are separate licenses for acupuncture, moxa treatment and herbal medicine. This type of specialization is fine but is inferior to Oriental Medicine as practiced in China and Korea today, where acupuncture and herbal medicine are combined for treatment. This rule can be applied to Korean pharmacists who prescribe and sell herbal medicines to patients. They do not pay much attention to the physical injuries of patients with blockage of Qi flow and this can cause disease. In these cases, their treatment becomes a temporary and symptomatic fix. If a patient's problem is more physical than internal, the pharmacist may have some serious moral and ethical problems.

Many people ask health food store and herbal shop employees to help them choose an herbal medicine. These people are not professionals in the field. Their understanding of herbal medicine is no better than yours. Pain and disease can interfere with your judgment and this is why you should always get advice from professionals.

THE FUTURE OF OREIENTAL MEDICINE IN THE UNITED STATES

Every medical practitioner should learn the acupuncture points in the human body in order to avoid injecting a hypodermic needle into an acupuncture point and causing severe pain and possibly Qi stagnation in that channel.

In June 1973, acupuncture anesthesia was first performed in the United States at the Naval Hospital in Portsmouth, Virginia. A 50 year-old woman suffered from a swollen throat and tongue which was blocking the air passage. The surgeons needed to make a hole through her throat in order to save her life, but because she had a weak heart and kidney trouble they were reluctant to use conventional anesthetics. I was asked to perform acupuncture anesthesia on her and the surgery was a success. I noticed that the patient felt fear and stress because she was awake during the surgery. This in itself was very psychologically painful to her. For this reason, I have reservations about the use of acupuncture alone for anesthesia. Even in China, acupuncture is combined during surgery with Western sedatives. The patient feels less physical pain, is calmer during surgery and recovers quicker.

Today the policy of the Chinese, Korean and Japanese governments on Oriental Medicine is to encourage the practitioners of Oriental Medicine to combine both Eastern and Western medicine and to research it with Western medical science. The problem is that there are not enough teachers in the field and one who studies both medicines will be a specialist in neither. Today in South Korea, practitioners of Eastern and Western medicine argue whether practitioners of Oriental Medicine should be allowed to use the stethoscope, to check blood pressure, order x-rays, blood tests or studies and compare prescriptions of Oriental and Western medicine. A step in the right direction is to allow practitioners of Oriental Medicine to study microbiology, biochemistry and basic diagnostic methods of Western medicine in the schools of Oriental Medicine in America.

In 1996, medical researchers found out that stomach ulcers and ulcerated colitis are caused by bacteria H-pylori and can be treated by antibiotics. Supposedly, antibiotics work equally well for everybody, as germ theory states in Western medicine. But each patient's level of physical and emotional stress is different and can cause different levels of stagnation of Qi flow according to Oriental Medicine theory. Someone with a severe physical injury or emotional stress has a less likely chance of being cured by antibiotics and even if a cure is achieved, the recurrence rate of the disease will be very high. Therefore, when treating any disease, we should always combine both Eastern and Western medicines for better results.

Human and animal sperm counts are declining every year as well as the sperm's potency. Deflation of the world's population is a possibility. Scientists blame this syndrome on pollution caused by industrialized countries. I have treated many couples for infertility. Most of the time, I restore the women's menstrual cycle and blood circulation in perfect condition. But if pregnancy still does not result, then I have the man get a sperm count. I recommend this practice to all acupuncturists. Having solved many infertility problems with many couples successfully, I believe Oriental Medicine will be the main tool to survival of the human race in the future.

Harvard Medical School researchers found out that after acupuncture treatment on the human body, endo opiate (endorphine) increases in the brain. It acts like a natural pain killer and may also be an important discovery in acupuncture theory. I have treated many patients with chronic sciatic pain. Usually one of their legs is colder and even thinner than the other. During and after acupuncture treatment their legs get stronger and warmer and their muscle tone improves. This kind of phenomenon cannot be explained by endorphine theory alone. Today there are a few universities and colleges that are doing acupuncture research. This research is mainly focused on hormonal, biochemical or physiological changes that can be observed after acupuncture treatment. I believe that their research should focus more on Qi flow and acupuncture channel theory in humans and animals.

Germ theory and antibiotics have been widely used to fight disease since the early twentieth century. What has been learned is that antibiotics cannot control many viruses and that many bacteria are developing resistance against most antibiotics. Genetic engineering is gaining in popularity but developing ways to fight disease will take time. I believe that a sophisticated measuring device will be developed to understand Qi flow in the human body which will greatly aid physicians in their battle against the diseases of mankind in the twenty first century.

The Myung Kim's Macro-Corelationism Theory

Specialization, separation and analysis in Western medicine has reached its limit with regard to diagnosis, prognosis and the treatment strategies for diseases. Modern Western medicine needs a new system and a new way of thinking. Western medical practitioners must learn to search for connectedness and the relationship of one disorder to another disorder. They must also check for many other factors as described in Chapter 4. The basis for diagnosis and prognosis which has been discussed throughout this book is what I refer to as the Macro-Corelationism Theory.

How to implement this theory? As described in this book, one should first survey and observe how one organ or part of one side of the body affects another organ or part in the same side of the body. Second, one should look for a psycho-somatic or soma-psychotic relationship of diseases as describe in Chapter 7, the Five Element Theory. Most recognize that an emotional problem can cause a physical problem. But we must also acknowledge that a physical disorder can affect the emotional well-being of a patient.

For Acupuncturists, it is time to understand and use the Myung Kim's Three Dimensional Four Inter-Channel Theory, time to realize and emphasize the importance of the Gall Bladder channel. For all other medical practitioners, it is time to understand the Myung Kim's Macro-Corelationism Theory and philosophy.

EPILOG

It is worthwhile to repeat the following items that appear earlier in this book for emphasis and clarification in the understanding of Oriental Medicine.

The science of Oriental Medicine is not as clear as Western medicine. Western medicine quantifies all matters and phenomena in the universe, which makes it easier to comprehend, whereas Oriental Medicine relies on feeling the flow of Qi, both in our bodies and the interaction of Qi in the universe. In addition, there are many conflicting theories of Oriental Medicine as Yin/Yang principles, and false information presented by commercialized translations of ancient texts and by self-appointed masters without the experience or the credentials.

The Western method of science relies on sight as a main measuring or quantifying device, or a "seeing is believing" philosophy. Yet before the invention of the electric tester, electricity existed in the universe. Similarly, there are many other unknown phenomena in the universe that we do not have devices to see or measure. This is why most people in the world today are skeptical about the existence of Qi flow in a human body.

But the abilities of man's sensory organs are limited, and creating devices to fit to our sense organs is thus limited as well. Our auditory ability is not as advanced as animals, who can hear low frequency sounds; our sight is not as refined as the owl, who can see at night, or the eagle, who can see at great distances.

Orientals, on the other hand, developed extraordinary senses through fasting meditation and Qi Gong practice instead of relying on sight alone or measuring devices like their Western counterparts. If we want to maximize our perceptual abilities to understand the universe, we should combine both the Eastern and Western cultures.

Human beings are always seeking a way to attain longevity without sickness, longevity with everlasting youth or everlasting youth with immortality. This has been true since homosapiens appeared on this planet Earth. Indian Yoga and Taoism philosophy and practice have helped some achieve these goals.

But any human being or living creature in this world will go through the inevitable path of life-birth, getting old, sickness and death, as in Buddha's teaching. Getting older means our organs are getting weaker, like an old car. Add to this the emotional and physical scars of life and, injuries to our bodies often without fully recovering from one injury to another.

Patients often ask "Can you cure this kind of disease or that kind of ailment?" If the patient's symptoms are severe and acute, the patient would probably have the specific tests and treatment, possibly emergency surgery, prescribed by Western doctors. But I recommend that everyone should check his or her body on a regular basis, much like Western doctors perform routine exams, to locate any abnormal feeling in the body, and then visit a Doctor of Oriental Medicine for an evaluation and diagnosis, before the symptoms became severe.

For example, a Western doctor would diagnosis a heart problem with an electrocardiogram and other specific measurements from tests. A Doctor of Oriental Medicine would ask if the patient had many dreams and nightmares, frightens easily, forgets easily, and experiences pain on the acupuncture points along the left-side Heart channel. Even without detecting heart palpitations, this patient would be diagnosed as Heart Qi deficient and/or Heart Qi Stagnation (see Chapter 12).

Another common question patients ask is "Do you have any good herbs to treat this or that disease?" The answer is yes, Oriental Medicine can provide herbal treatments like Western pharmaceutical medicine. However, before you take any herbs, you should be diagnosed by a Doctor of Oriental Medicine so that you get herbs for your unique condition.

For example, if you have a cold, you could go to the corner drug store and buy common cold medicine. Or you could go to a doctor or Oriental Medicine, to see if you have "wind cold" - runny nose, chills, sneezing and coughing white phlegm, or a "wind heat" cold - dry nose, sore throat, mild fever, coughing and yellow phlegm. Another example is the herb Asian ginseng root, which has become very popular in America. But this herb is not good for people with warm body types. It is suitable for older people who have lethargy, low sexual energy, and a constant feeling of coldness (Yang deficiency).

Not only does herbal medicine have Western medicine-like properties, such as digestive, sedative, anti-biotic, diuretic and laxative, but it also has tonification properties, can build Qi energy, produce blood and balance Yin and Yang — things which cannot be done with the Western medicine.

"How many Acupuncture treatments are needed? Should I combine them with herbal medicine? What should be the ratio between the two treatments?" If you have more physical problems than internal organ problems, then take more acupuncture treatments than herbal medicine. If you have more organ problems than physical problems, then take more herbal medicine than acupuncture treatments.

We have seen throughout this book that Oriental Medicine is an excellent tool for preventing disease, treating chronic illness and maintaining good health. In fact you can have acupuncture treatments, take herbs, and practice Qi Gong on a regular basis, as long as you adjust your treatments according to the Yin/Yang principle. Western medicine, by contrast, is excellent for treating acute diseases, detecting infections, treating epidemics, treating diseases, treating emergency situations and for performing surgery.

When you receive treatment for any disease, even cancer or AIDS, try as many methods as possible: acupuncture, moxa, cupping, Qi Gong massage, Qi Gong practice, meditation and even prayer as described in Chapter 9.

Western medicine cannot stimulate or strengthen each organ function as Oriental Medicine can, especially when combined with acupuncture, moxa, massage and Qi Gong.

Who does not have any emotional or physical scars and injuries? Who has lived a lifetime without any imbalance of Yin and Yang, Qi and Blood deficiency or stagnation in this world today?

I like to advise anyone who wants to live without sickness, attain longevity and everlasting youth, as a Taoist wishes, to check with a Doctor of Oriental Medicine at least once a month, or once a week or even once a day, like kings and aristocracy of the Orient did not too long ago, and well-known actors living in Hollywood do today. Because Oriental Medicine is an excellent tool for promoting good health, you can have acupuncture treatments or herbal medicine as often as you like, just like you can get a massage at any time. You do not have to be sick to benefit from Oriental Medicine.

You should go to a Doctor of Oriental Medicine who has licenses in both acupuncture and herbal medicine. Make sure you check licenses, even if the herbalist claims to have learned from a father or grandfather. An incorrect herbal medication can have a harmful effect on your body, or provide a temporary fix, much like Western pharmaceutical medicine. The physical injuries that are prevalent to Western people, such as those caused by sports, car accidents and surgery scars, need to be checked and treated for blocked acupuncture channels, not by herbal treatments alone.

Last spring, I gave a seminar at an acupuncture school in New England. I noticed a survey of the most commonly used acupuncture points. Of the points listed, only one point came from the Gall Bladder Channel. It was the least popular of all the points on the survey. I believe that this is true of most acupuncture styles in the world today.

I have treated more than twenty patients today. More than seventy-five percent of them had Gall Bladder channel problems.

2 patients had gall stones.

3 patients had back pain which radiated down to the Gall Bladder channel.

1 patient had hair loss related to a Gall Bladder channel problem.

2 patients had prostate problems.

1 patient had hepatitis.

2 patients had ovarian and uterine tumors.

1 patient had a brain tumor

2 patients had breast cancer which had been removed surgically.

1 patient had lower back pain, knee and testicle problems.

1 patient was impotent.

Most of their disorders started from lower back pain. Some patients showed eye and ear problems and vertigo. Some patients showed a combination of Gall Bladder channel problems with neck pain that radiated down to the Small Intestine channel to cause carpal tunnel syndrome.

Oriental medical theory indicates that a disorder can manifest itself different ways in each patient. This is in contrast to Western medicine which recognizes only a few standard symptoms.

It is unusual to write my own interpretations of my own book. I am doing so to help you the reader understand not only each part of this book but also the entire text.

I have discussed politics and my personal experiences on escaping from North Korea, martial arts, the Korean and Viet Nam wars in the beginning of this book to demonstrate that my life is living proof of Taoism philosophy; Yin and Yang.

While I have experienced hardship throughout my life, I developed medicine instead of weapons. I do not hate Japanese, Chinese, Russian or American people. I proved this with my medical career. I always try to love and harmonize with everything in the universe, even empty space, just as in Oriental paintings. I can appreciate the beauty, capacity for imagination and feeling of nothingness.

It is frequently reported that some cancer and heart disease rates are declining today due to advances in research and better methods of early detection. No doubt this is true but perhaps another contributing factor is that more and more people - as much as 1/3 of the U.S. population - are being treated with Oriental Medicine on a regular basis. I am sure that this is playing an unrecognized role in the improvement of people's health as well, but you don't read that in the newspaper.

I have read about some new cancer research data in the *Boston Globe* newspaper. A Harvard medical team found out that American's cancer rate is two percent traceable to environmental pollution, ten percent to genetics and seventy percent of cancer occurrences are caused by ciga-rettes, alcohol, poor diet, and obesity.

I would like to advise the medical team to turn their heads away from their microscopes and computer screens, which cause blurry vision and nearsightedness. Try to look at the entire patient. Look over your school fence; my clinic is located just two miles from your school. Finally, look even further over the Pacific Ocean, where the Oriental culture is.

November 22, 1996 at Cambridge, Massachusetts

Myung Chill Kim

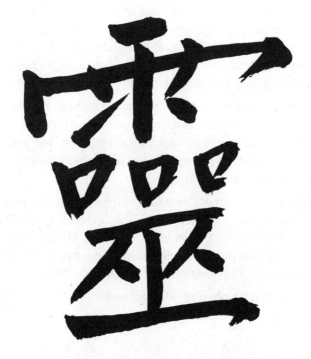

**LING
(SPIRIT OF DEAD)**

Resources
National Commission for the Certification of Acupuncturists (N.C.C.A.)
1424, 16th Street, N.W. Suite 501
Washington, D.C. 20036
(202) 232-1404 Phone, (202) 462-6157 Fax

Council of Colleges of Acupuncture and Oriental Medicine (C.C.A.O.M.)
8403 Colesville Road, Suite 370
Silver Spring, MD 20910
(301) 608-9175 Phone, (301) 608-9576 Fax

Request for C.C.A.O.M. member school brochure or catalog packet:
Package of college brochures - $15.00
Package of colleges catalogs - $50.00

For information on services and products, contact:
Myung Kim's Acupuncture and Herbal Clinic
Mailing Address:
PO Box 577, Belmont, MA 02178

Bibliography
English

The Yellow Emperor's Classics of Internal Medicine
ILZA VEITH, 1949 University of California Press

Chinese Herbal Medicine Materia Medica
Dan Bensky and Andrew Gamble 1986 Eastland Press

Essentials of Chinese Acupuncture
1979 Beijing Foreign Languages Press

ACUPUNCTURE A Comprehensive Text
1981 Eastland Press

The Web that has no Weaver - Understanding Chinese Medicine
Ted J. Kaptchuk, 1983 Congdon and Weed Inc.

ACUPUNCTURE
Felix Mann MB , 1962 Vintage Books Edition

Traditional Medicine in Modern China
Crozier, 1968 Harvard University Press

China, A General Survey
1982 Beijing Foreign Languages Press

Chen's History of Chinese Medical History
Hsu, 1977 Modern Drug Publisher, Taipei, China

Making of a Peasant Doctor
Hsiao, 1976 Beijing Foreign Languages Press

Handbook of Chinese Herbs and Formulas Volume I & II
Him Che Yeung O.M.D Ph.D., 1983

Culture and Healing in Asian Societies
Kleinman, 1978 Schenkman Publishers

Modern China and Traditional Chinese Medicine
Risse, 1968 Thomas Publishers

Acupuncture for Self Defense
Myung Chill Kim, 1973 T.K.D. Publication

KOREAN
Huang Je Nae Kyung (Yellow Emperor's Internal Medicine)
1955, Dong Yang Press

Huang Je Nae Kyung (Yellow Emperor's Internal Medicine)
1961, Soo Su Won Publication

Huang Je Nae Kyung (Yellow Emperor's Internal Medicine)
1975 Dong Bang Press

Huang Je Nae Kyung (Yellow Emperor's Internal Medicine)
1983 Sung Bo Sa

Huang Je Nae Kyung (Yellow Emperor's Internal Medicine)
1994 Translated by Lee Kyung Woo, Yue Kang Press

Huang Je Nae Kyung Woon Gi Hae Suk (Yellow Emperor's Internal Medicine - Qi Circulation) 1975 Translated by Back Won Gi, Ko Mu Sa

Bon Cho Hak (Chinese Materia Medica)
1968 Dong Yang Press

Bon Cho Hak (Chinese Materia Medica)
1975 Translated by Lee Sang Yin, Soo Su Sa Press

Sang Han Lun (Treatise on Cold Induced Disease)
Translated by Che Yin Sik, 1971 Ko Mun Sa Press

Won Byung Lun (Treatise on Heat Induced Disease)
1990 Sam Sup Choi, Sung Bo Sa

Sa Sang Che Jil (Four Type Constitutional Acupuncture)
1890 Je Ma Lee

Dong Yi Bo Gam (Great Collection of Oriental Medicine)
1602 Hue Jun

Dong Yi Bo Gam (Great Collection of Oriental Medicine)
1979 Min Chang Sa

Sa Am Do In Chim Gu Hak (Sa Am Method of Acupuncture)
1575 Sa Am Do In

Sa Am Chim Bup (Sa Am Method of Acupuncture)
1975 Cho Se Hyung, Sung Bo Sa

Joong Yi Nae Kwa (Traditional Chinese Internal Medicine)
1959 Dong Yang Press

Joong Yi Bu Yin Kwa (Traditional Chinese Internal Medicine - Gynecology)
1963 Dong Yang Press

Joong Yi So A Kwa (Traditional Chinese Internal Medicine - Pediatrics)
1965 Dong Yang Press

Chun Yun Yak Mul Dae Sa Jun (Illustrated Natural Medicine Encyclopedia)
Kim Jae Woo, 1984 Nam San Dang Press

CHINESE
*Huang Di Nei Jing Su Wen (Yellow Emperor's Internal Medicine and Simple
Questions)* Beijing, 1963 People's Press

Nan Jing (Classic of Difficulties)
1650 Xu Lingtai

Zhen Jiu Dacheng (Great Compendium of Acupuncture and Moxibustion)
Yang Ji Zhou 1601

Shisi Jing Hahui (Elucidation of the Fourteen Channels)
Yuan Hua Shou 1341

Jingui Yaolue Fang Lun (Prescription from the Golden Casket)
Zhang Zhong Jing 220

Furen Da Quan Liang Fang (Great Collection of Prescriptions for Women)
Chen Zi Ming 1237

Zen Jiu Da Quan (Acupuncture and Moxibustion)
Xu Feng 1439

Bencao Congxin (New Edition of Pharmacopia)
Wu Yiluo 1757

Qijing Bamai Kao (Eight Miscellaneous Channels)
Li Shizhen 1578

Xin Bian Yaowu Xue (New Edition of Pharmacology)
Chen XinQian 1974 People's Health Publishing Company

Zhong Yao Da Ci Dian (Great Dictionary of Chinese Medicine)
1977 Shanghai Science Publishing Co.

Zhongguo Yixue Shilue (Brief History of Chinese Medicine)
Jia De Dao, 1979 Shanxi People's Publishing Co.

Shiyong Zhong Yi Xue (Practical Chinese Medicine)
1977 Sichuan People's Press

Ben Cao Yan Yi (Materia Medica)
Kou Zhong Shi 1116

Ben Cao Bei Yao (Materia Medica)
Wang Ang 1751

Shang Han Lun (Treatise on Cold Induced Disease)
Zhang Zhong Jing 169

Wen Bing Lun (Treatise on Heat Induced Disease)
Ye Tien Si 1260

Index

Glossary

1 Taoist - The Chinese term Tao is usually translated as "The Way" in the sense of a path. It also can be understood as the unity of all things which is divided into Yin and Yang. So our wandering physician here is following his path to the Tao. Taoist philosophy is perhaps the most important influence on Chinese medicine. Lao Tzu and Chuang Tzu are the most widely known Taoist writers if you are interested in learning more, but keep in mind that Lao Tzu wrote "The Tao that can be told of is not the eternal Tao."

2 Qi - This will be discussed in Chapter 2.

3 Ninja - In 16th and 17th Century feudal Japan, the Ninjas were spies and assassins trained in martial techniques that had come to Japan from China via Korea.

4 Kidney 1 - See the Kidney section of Chapter 10.

5 Pericardium 8 - See the Pericardium section of Chapter 10.

6 Moxa - The use of dried mugwort leaves (Folium artemisia argyi) in moxibustion is discussed in Chapter 9.

7 Urinary Bladder 21 - See the Urinary Bladder section of Chapter 10.

8 Back Shu points are explained in Chapter 10.

9 Large Intestine 4 - See the Large Intestine section of Chapter 10.

10 Liver 3 - See the Liver section of Chapter 10.

11 Qi Gong-An internal style martial art. Can also be practiced as a slow breathing exercise or as a form of meditation to cultivate Qi energy.

12 Tai Chi-Another internal style martial art which uses slow breathing and slow movement as a means of cultivating Qi.

13 DNA - Deoxyribonucleic acid is an organic molecule that resides in the nucleus of each cell and contains the organism's genetic information.

14 Spleen - See the Spleen section of Chapter 12 for a discussion of the spleen in Western and Eastern medicine.

15 Shen - See the Heart section of Chapter 12.

16 Hun - See the Heart section of Chapter 12.

17 Po - See the Heart section of Chapter 12.

18 Ling - See the Heart section of Chapter 12.

19 Cha Ryuk - This is a Korean hard style Qi Gong that has similarities to martial arts. In addition to meditation, the breath is held for long periods and the chest and abdomen are struck with the fist.

20 UB 10 - See the last section of Chapter 10.

21 UB 11 - See the last section of Chapter 10.

22 Spirit possession-See the Heart section of Chapter 12.

23 I Ching - See Figures 6-5 and 6-6 in Chapter 6 and Figure 10-32 in Chapter 10.

24 Lao Tzu - This legendary figure, who may have lived between 604-531 B.C.E and whose name means "Old Master", is credited with being the founder of Taoism.

25 Tao Te Ching - The classic book of Taoist philosophy. Often translated as The Way of Life.

26 Buddhism - Religion founded on the teachings of Gautama Buddha, an Indian sage thought to have lived in the sixth century B.C.E.

27 Ayurvedic Medicine - The traditional medicine of India, which uses herbs and massage to treat patients.

28 Bhagavad Gita - This section of the Indian epic Mahabharata is a dialogue between Krishna and Prince Arjuna which presents the ideas of action without attachment also found in Tao Te Ching.

29 Cupping - See Chapter 9.

30 Phenotype - The physical appearance of an organism.

31 Genotype - The genetic makeup of an organism.

32 St. Patrick's Day-Held on March 17 in honor of St. Patrick, the patron saint of Ireland.

33 Middle Jiao - See the end of Chapter 10 (channel theory) for note on Triple Warmer.

34 Asi point - Any point on the skin where finger pressure may cause pain other than the common acupuncture points.

35 David Bohm (1916-1993) was a theoretical physicist at Birkbeck College, London, and the author of Quantum Physics (1951). His understanding of the nature of the universe was influenced not only by his deep understanding of physics but also by his training in Indian yoga.

36 All but one of the acupuncture channels have names which correspond to organs in the body. The exception, of course, is the Sanjiao Channel, which is translated as Triple Burner, Triple Heater, or Triple Warmer depending on the translator. But what is it? Is it another organ or something else entirely?

The traditional explanation is that the Triple Warmer refers to the trunk of the body. Using this approach, the body can be divided into three regions. The Upper Warmer corresponds to the Heart and Lungs, the Middle Warmer to the Spleen and Stomach, and the Lower Warmer to the Kidney and Urinary Bladder. Different acupuncture and herbal treatments target different Warmers depending upon the patient's presentation.

The Back Shu and Front Mu points of most organs are located near their corresponding organ. Taking into account the locations of the Triple Warmer Back Shu (UB 22) and Front Mu (REN 5) points, many people have suggested that the Triple Warmer is the pancreas, an important organ which has no channel associated with it. Among the functions of the Yang organs are digestion and transformation of food and the transportation of nutrients and wastes. The pancreas secretes pancreatic juice which helps to digest proteins, fats, and starches. It also houses the Isles of Langerhans, endocrine glands which secrete the hormones glucagon and insulin, which regulate the levels of glucose in the blood. From these functions it is easy to see why some people have wanted to consider the pancreas and the Triple Warmer the same Yang organ with different names.

Some acupuncturists have recently been considering another definition for the Triple Warmer. Perhaps it is actually the endocrine system, more specifically the pineal and pituitary glands and the hypothalamus, all located in the brain. This first occurred to me when I considered the pathway of the Triple Warmer Channel, which runs into the ear and could connect internally to these glands in the brain. The pineal gland, which is sometimes called the third eye because it is influenced by the amount of light entering the eyes, secretes melatonin which is thought to regulate the body's circadian rhythms and other cycles. The pituitary gland is often called the master gland of the body. It secretes nine major hormones with a wide variety of functions, including the regulation of growth, the activities of other endocrine glands, and the induction of labor. The hypothalamus is not a gland but the part of the brain to which the pituitary gland is connected. It regulates the release of hormones from the pituitary gland and also controls many body functions that are related to homeostasis, such as temperature, appetite and thirst.

37 Cun - This is a unit of measurement which will be discussed in the Proportional Measurements section of this chapter.

38 Refer to the Liver Qi stagnation section of Chapter 12.

39 The belt channel consists of GB 26, 27, and 28. It is the part of the gall bladder channel where Qi circulates around the waistline as a belt. The belt channel is one of eight extra channels besides the 12 regular channels that move through our hands, feet, and throughout our body. The du (governing) and ren (conceptual) channels are two of these eight extra channels.

40 False Heat - Tidal heat or afternoon heat. See Yin Deficiency Syndrome in the last section of Chapter 8.

41 Ginger moxa - When applying moxa directly on skin, use a slice of ginger to protect the skin. Take a slice of ginger about 3mm or 1/8 inch thickness and make small holes in it. Place it on the skin, then place the moxa on the ginger and light it.

Order Form

Myung Kim Acupuncture, Chi Gong, Herb Clinic   :178
6444 NW Expressway, Suite 420D
Oklahoma City, OK 73132
(405) 470-7131
masterkim@myungchillkim.com

AVAILABLE BOOKS BY MYUNG CHILL KIM:
Oriental Medicine and Cancer ($19.95)

UPCOMING BOOKS BY MYUNG CHILL KIM:
Qi Gong   (SPRING 1998)
Oriental Herbal Medicine (Fall 1998)

(PRINT OR TYPE THE FOLLOWING INFORMATION)

Company Name:_____

Name:_____

Address:_____

City:_____ State:_____ Zip:_____

Telephone:__(   )_____

SALES TAX:
Please add 5% for books shipped to a Massachusetts address.

SHIPPING:
Air Mail: $3.50 per book

Book Rate: $2.00 for the first book and 75¢ for each additional book
Allow three to four weeks for delivery

PAYMENT METHOD:
( ) Check   ( ) Money Order   ( ) Visa
( ) MasterCard   ( ) American Express ( ) Discover

Card Number: _____Expiration Date: _____

Name on Card: _____

Total Order: _____

MA Sales Tax (5%) _____(Massachusetts Residence Only)

Shipping: _____

Order Form

S
Myung Kim Acupuncture, Chi Gong, Herb Clinic
6444 NW Expressway, Suite 420D
Oklahoma City, OK 73132
(405) 470-7131
masterkim@myungchillkim.com

Available books by Myung Chill Kim:
Oriental Medicine and Cancer ($19.95)

Upcoming books by Myung Chill Kim:
Qi Gong   (SPRING 1998)
Oriental Herbal Medicine (Fall 1998)

(PRINT OR TYPE THE FOLLOWING INFORMATION)

Company Name: _____

Name: _____

Address: _____

City:_____ State:_____ Zip:_____

Telephone:___(   )_____

Sales Tax:
Please add 5% for books shipped to a Massachusetts address.

Shipping:
Air Mail: $3.50 per book

Book Rate: $2.00 for the first book and 75¢ for each additional book
Allow three to four weeks for delivery

Payment Method:
( ) Check   ( ) Money Order   ( ) Visa
( ) MasterCard   ( ) American Express ( ) Discover

Card Number: _____Expiration Date: _____

Name on Card: _____

Total Order: _____

MA Sales Tax (5%) _____(Massachusetts Residence Only)

Shipping: _____